Makeup Tutorial for Black Women.
Makeup Mastery for Beginners

Essential Techniques, Skin Care, Secrets, and Beauty Tips to Unleash Your True Glow

Nala Johnson

Table of Content

Introduction:

Welcome

Welcome to "Makeup Tutorial for Black Women: Makeup Mastery for Beginners." This book is a celebration of you—your skin, your heritage, and your unique beauty. As you embark on this journey into the world of makeup, we invite you to explore the boundless possibilities that makeup offers to enhance and express your individuality.

Whether you're picking up a makeup brush for the first time or you're looking to refine your existing skills, this guide is designed with you in mind. We understand that stepping into the diverse world of beauty products can be overwhelming, which is why we have tailored this book to make your experience both enlightening and enjoyable.

Makeup should be empowering, a way to express who you are on the inside by enhancing what's on the outside. Our goal is to provide you with the tools and knowledge necessary to navigate the makeup aisle with confidence, to make informed choices about the products you use, and to apply makeup in a way that truly reflects and respects your individual beauty.

This book will serve as your personal makeup consultant, guiding you through each step of your makeup application process. From understanding the basics of skin care to mastering the art of makeup application, we cover it all. With each chapter, you'll gain both the confidence and the skills needed to enhance your natural beauty and unleash your true glow.

So, open these pages with excitement and readiness to embark on a transformative journey. We are thrilled to be part of your adventure in discovering and mastering makeup techniques that celebrate and illuminate your black beauty. Welcome, let's begin this beautiful transformation together.

Understanding Your Skin

Embarking on your makeup journey begins with a fundamental understanding of your skin—its type, texture, and tone. Your skin is as unique as you are, and understanding its specific characteristics is crucial for selecting makeup and skincare products that enhance rather than mask your natural beauty.

This section is devoted to helping you discern not only your skin type—be it oily, dry, combination, or sensitive—but also the nuances that come with having melanin-rich skin. We'll explore how different skin types can affect your overall makeup application and longevity, how to address common concerns such as hyperpigmentation and uneven skin tone, and how to choose products that truly suit and benefit your skin.

For black women, skincare can sometimes be challenging, as the market has historically underrepresented darker skin tones. However, armed with the right knowledge, you can make empowered choices that lead to healthy and glowing skin. We will delve into the science behind why certain ingredients are beneficial or harmful, helping you to curate a skincare routine that addresses your specific needs.

Understanding your skin also involves recognizing the importance of sun protection, hydration, and proper diet—all of which play significant roles in skin health. We'll provide practical tips and techniques for maintaining the health of your skin through lifestyle choices, as well as through topical treatments.

Armed with a deeper knowledge of your skin's needs, you'll be better prepared to navigate the vast world of beauty products. This will not only improve your makeup application but also ensure that your skin remains vibrant and healthy beneath the makeup.

Through this exploration, our hope is for you to become more attuned to your skin's unique voice, making every makeup choice an informed and beneficial decision. Let's begin this foundational journey together, paving the way for a skincare and makeup routine that celebrates and cares for your distinctive beauty.

The Importance of Makeup for Every Shade

Makeup is an incredible tool for self-expression and creativity. It has the power to transform not just how we look, but how we feel about ourselves. For black women, makeup serves an even more profound role—it is a celebration of cultural identity and individual beauty across a spectrum of shades. In this section, we dive into why makeup is so vital for every shade, especially for those often underrepresented in the beauty industry.

For many years, the range of products available on the market did not fully cater to the rich diversity of dark skin tones. This lack of inclusivity not only made it challenging to find suitable makeup options but also subtly implied that beauty was a monolithic standard. Today, we are witnessing a positive shift towards a more inclusive approach in beauty, where every skin tone is celebrated and catered to. This book aims to be part of that change by ensuring you find makeup that not only matches but also enhances your skin.

Understanding the importance of makeup for every shade means recognizing that each shade requires different formulations, pigments, and care. Makeup should complement your skin, enriching its natural tone without masking it. This involves choosing the right foundation that seamlessly blends with your skin, eyeshadows that enhance your natural eye color, and lipsticks that make your smile pop.

Moreover, makeup is a tool for empowerment. It allows you to take control of your image and present yourself to the world in a way that feels true to you. Whether it's a bold, dramatic look for a night out or a simple, subtle application for everyday wear, makeup can boost your confidence and allow you to fully express your personality.

In this book, we'll explore how to select and apply makeup that not only suits your skin tone but also supports your vision of personal beauty. We will provide you with the techniques, tips, and guidance needed to navigate the colorful world of makeup, ensuring that you feel represented, respected, and radiant.

Ultimately, makeup is more than just color applied to the face—it's an art form and a form of personal storytelling. Let's embrace this art together, celebrating the richness of your shade with every brush stroke.

Chapter 1: Skin Care Fundamentals

Understanding Your Skin Type

The first and perhaps most crucial step in building a skincare routine is accurately identifying your skin type. This foundational knowledge enables you to select the best products and techniques suited to your skin's unique needs, ensuring you care for it most effectively.

Types of Skin

Typically, skin is classified into five main types:

1. **Normal:** This skin type is well-balanced, neither too oily nor too dry, and has few imperfections or sensitivity issues.

2. **Oily:** Characterized by an excess production of sebum, oily skin often appears shiny, with larger pores and is more prone to acne and breakouts.
3. **Dry:** Dry skin can feel tight and rough and appear dull due to a lack of moisture and natural oils. It may also flake or become irritated more easily.
4. **Combination:** Combination skin features two or more different skin types on the face, typically with oiliness in the T-zone (forehead, nose, and chin) and normal to dry skin on other parts of the face.
5. **Sensitive:** Sensitive skin is prone to itching, burning, and redness and can react adversely to certain skincare products and environmental factors.

Determining Your Skin Type

To determine your skin type, you can perform a simple test at home:

- **Cleanse your face** thoroughly with a gentle cleanser and pat it dry. Leave your skin bare (without applying any additional skincare products) and wait for about an hour.
- After an hour, examine your skin in a mirror, paying close attention to any shine on your forehead, nose, cheeks, and chin.
- Press a clean tissue against different areas of your face. If oil appears on the tissue from the forehead, nose, and chin, it suggests oily or combination skin. No oil suggests normal or dry skin.

Importance for Black Skin

For black women, knowing your skin type is especially important as certain skin types may be more prone to specific conditions like hyperpigmentation or keloid scarring. Oily skin types, which are common among black women, may struggle with post-inflammatory hyperpigmentation (PIH), where acne or even minor injuries can lead to dark spots. Dry skin may appear ashy if not moisturized adequately.

Tailoring Your Skincare

Once your skin type is determined, you can tailor your skincare regimen to address its specific needs and challenges. For example:

- **Oily skin** benefits from lightweight, water-based products and regular exfoliation to keep pores clear and reduce excess oil.
- **Dry skin** requires rich, emollient creams that hydrate and seal in moisture to combat dryness and flaking.
- **Sensitive skin** needs hypoallergenic, fragrance-free products to minimize the risk of irritation.

Understanding your skin type is the first step toward healthier, more radiant skin. With this knowledge, you'll be equipped to choose the right products and establish a skincare routine that brings out the best in your skin, enhancing its natural beauty and addressing any specific issues you may face.

The Basics of a Good Skin Care Routine

A well-structured skincare routine is essential for maintaining healthy, radiant skin. For beginners, especially those with dark skin tones, understanding the basic steps of effective skincare can make a significant difference in skin appearance and health. This section will guide you through the foundational elements of a daily skincare regimen tailored to the unique needs of black skin.

Step 1: Cleansing

Cleansing is the first step in any skincare routine. It removes dirt, oil, and impurities from the skin's surface and prepares it for further treatments. For those with dark skin, which may be more prone to hyperpigmentation, using a gentle cleanser can prevent irritation that might lead to discoloration. It's important to cleanse twice a day, morning and night, to ensure that the skin remains clean and vibrant.

Step 2: Toning

Toning is a crucial step that often gets overlooked. A good toner can help restore the skin's pH balance, remove residual dirt or makeup left after cleansing, and tighten the pores. For black skin, look for toners that contain ingredients like glycolic acid or salicylic acid to help manage oil production and prevent breakouts, without over-drying the skin.

Step 3: Moisturizing

Moisturizing hydrates the skin and locks in moisture, which is vital for all skin types but especially for dry or mature skin, which can appear ashy if neglected. Moisturizers for dark skin should be rich in hydrating ingredients such as hyaluronic acid, glycerin, or natural oils. Even oily skin needs moisturization; opt for light, non-comedogenic formulas that hydrate without clogging pores.

Step 4: Sun Protection

Sun protection is critical for all skin types, but it is particularly important for black skin due to the common misconception that melanin alone provides enough protection against UV rays. Daily use of a broad-spectrum SPF of at least 30 can help prevent premature aging and protect against the development of dark spots and skin cancer. Choose sunscreens that do not leave a white cast and are designed to blend seamlessly into darker skin tones.

Additional Steps: Exfoliation and Treatment

- **Exfoliation:** Regular exfoliation, about 1-2 times a week, is beneficial for removing dead skin cells and promoting cell turnover. For black skin, chemical exfoliants like alpha hydroxy acids (AHAs) or beta hydroxy acids (BHAs) are preferred over harsh scrubs, as they are less likely to cause irritation or exacerbate hyperpigmentation.
- **Treatment Products:** If you have specific skin concerns, such as acne, dark spots, or fine lines, incorporating targeted treatment products like serums or spot treatments can be beneficial. Choose products with active ingredients that target your concerns while being mindful of their potency to avoid irritation.

By following these essential steps, you can establish a skincare routine that not only maintains the health of your skin but also enhances its natural beauty. Each step is designed to address the particular needs and challenges of black skin, ensuring that you provide the best care possible for your unique complexion.

Special Considerations for Black Skin

While the basics of skincare apply to everyone, black skin has unique characteristics and needs that require special attention. This section will explore these specific considerations, helping you to tailor your skincare regimen to better suit the particular demands of melanin-rich skin.

Hyperpigmentation

One of the most common concerns for black skin is hyperpigmentation. This occurs when excess melanin forms deposits in the skin, often as a result of inflammation, sun exposure, acne, or irritation. To manage and prevent hyperpigmentation, incorporate products that contain ingredients like vitamin C, niacinamide, and retinoids, which are known for their brightening properties and ability to even out skin tone. Additionally, consistent use of sunscreen is crucial to prevent dark spots from becoming darker.

Keloids

Black skin is more prone to developing keloids, which are raised scars that form at the site of skin injury. Preventing keloids begins with minimizing skin trauma—be gentle when handling your skin, especially if you are acne-prone. If you are susceptible to keloids, consider discussing preventive treatments with a dermatologist, especially when considering procedures like piercings or tattooing.

Dryness and Ashiness

Due to its texture and makeup, black skin can often appear dry or ashy if not properly moisturized. To combat this, use rich, emollient creams and butters that contain ingredients like shea butter, cocoa butter, and oils like coconut or jojoba. These ingredients provide deep hydration and help to seal in moisture, giving the skin a healthy, radiant glow.

Sebum Production

Black skin often produces more sebum, which can lead to a shiny appearance and the development of acne. It's important to balance the skin's oil production without stripping it of its natural oils. Opt for lightweight, water-based moisturizers, and use non-comedogenic products that won't clog pores. Incorporating a gentle, regular exfoliation routine can also help manage excess oil and prevent acne.

Sun Protection

There is a common myth that black skin does not need sunscreen due to the natural protection offered by melanin. However, while melanin does provide some protection against UV radiation, it is not enough to prevent skin damage. Sunscreen is essential for protecting against sunburn, reducing the risk of skin cancer, and preventing the uneven darkening of hyperpigmented areas. Look for broad-spectrum sunscreens that are lightweight and don't leave a white residue.

By considering these specific needs, you can create a skincare routine that not only addresses the general requirements of keeping skin healthy and hydrated but also tackles the unique challenges faced by black skin. This tailored approach ensures that your skin not only looks its best but is also resilient and well-cared for in the long term.

Product Recommendations

Choosing the right skincare products is crucial for maintaining healthy, radiant skin, especially for black skin which may have specific needs and concerns. This section provides carefully curated product recommendations to help you build an effective skincare routine tailored to the unique characteristics of black skin.

Cleansers

Gentle Foaming Cleanser: Ideal for removing excess oil without stripping the skin of its natural moisture. Look for products that contain ingredients like glycerin or hyaluronic acid.

- Recommended Product: CeraVe Foaming Facial Cleanser

Cream-Based Cleanser: Best for dry or sensitive skin, as it hydrates while it cleanses.

- Recommended Product: La Roche-Posay Toleriane Hydrating Gentle Cleanser

Toners

Hydrating Toner: Aids in restoring the skin's pH balance and provides an extra layer of moisture. Ingredients like rose water or chamomile are excellent for soothing the skin.

- Recommended Product: Thayers Alcohol-Free Rose Petal Witch Hazel Facial Toner

Exfoliating Toner: Contains AHAs or BHAs to help reduce the appearance of large pores and control oil production.

- Recommended Product: The Ordinary Glycolic Acid 7% Toning Solution

Moisturizers

For Oily Skin: Lightweight, gel-based moisturizers that hydrate without adding excess oil.

- Recommended Product: Neutrogena Hydro Boost Water Gel

For Dry Skin: Rich creams that contain emollients to lock in moisture, ideal for preventing ashiness.

- Recommended Product: CeraVe Moisturizing Cream

Sunscreens

Broad-Spectrum SPF: A must-have to protect against UVA and UVB rays, look for formulas that blend well into dark skin without leaving a white cast.

- Recommended Product: Black Girl Sunscreen SPF 30

Treatments for Hyperpigmentation

Serums with Vitamin C or Retinoids: Effective for fading dark spots and evening out skin tone.

- Recommended Product: Paula's Choice C15 Super Booster

Brightening Creams: Targeted treatments that help reduce hyperpigmentation and enhance skin radiance.

- Recommended Product: Ambi Fade Cream

Specialty Items

Exfoliants: Products containing salicylic acid or mandelic acid are great for gentle exfoliation and are effective in treating and preventing acne.

- Recommended Product: Drunk Elephant T.L.C. Framboos Glycolic Night Serum

Face Masks: Clay masks for oil control and hydration masks for dry skin can be used weekly to address specific skin concerns.

- Recommended Product: Aztec Secret Indian Healing Clay

By integrating these products into your skincare regimen, you can address the unique concerns associated with black skin, such as oil control, moisture retention, and hyperpigmentation management. Always remember to patch test new products and gradually introduce them into your routine to see how your skin reacts. This personalized approach ensures your skincare is both effective and harmonious with your skin's needs.

Chapter 2: Skin Prep for Makeup

Proper skin preparation is a critical step in achieving flawless makeup application, particularly for black skin, which may have unique concerns such as hyperpigmentation and uneven skin tone. This chapter delves into how to effectively prepare your skin for makeup, ensuring a smooth canvas that enhances your natural beauty.

Importance of Hydration

Hydration is a cornerstone of healthy skin and is essential for achieving a flawless makeup application. Well-hydrated skin not only looks more plump and vibrant but also provides a smooth base for makeup, helping to ensure that it applies evenly and lasts longer. Here we explore why hydration is crucial for skin health, particularly for black skin, and how to effectively hydrate before makeup application.

Why Hydration Matters

Hydrated skin results from adequate water content both inside and out, which helps maintain skin elasticity, reduce the appearance of fine lines, and allow for seamless makeup application. For black skin, which may be more prone to dryness and ashiness, maintaining hydration can enhance the skin's natural glow and prevent the makeup from looking flaky or patchy.

Internal Hydration

- **Drinking Water:** The simplest and most effective way to hydrate your skin is by drinking plenty of water throughout the day. Aim for at least 8 glasses a day, more if you are active or live in a dry climate.
- **Diet:** Incorporating water-rich foods into your diet, such as cucumbers, oranges, watermelons, and celery, can also help increase your overall hydration levels.

External Hydration

- **Moisturizers:** Applying a daily moisturizer suitable for your skin type is crucial. For oily skin, choose a lightweight, non-comedogenic moisturizer that hydrates without adding excess oil. For dry skin, a richer, emollient-based moisturizer can help lock in moisture.
- **Hyaluronic Acid:** This powerhouse ingredient can attract and retain moisture from the atmosphere into your skin, making it a valuable addition to your

skincare routine. Use a serum or moisturizer that lists hyaluronic acid as one of the top ingredients.
- **Hydrating Primers:** Before makeup application, using a hydrating primer can significantly improve the longevity and appearance of your makeup. It acts as a protective barrier between your skin and makeup, locking in moisture and smoothing out the skin's texture.

Pre-Makeup Hydration Tips

- **Cleansing Gently:** Start with a gentle cleanser to remove impurities without stripping the skin of its natural oils.
- **Layering Products:** After cleansing, apply a hydrating serum followed by a moisturizer. Allow each product to absorb fully before applying the next layer. This layering technique ensures maximum hydration without leaving the skin feeling greasy.
- **Refreshing Sprays:** Throughout the day, especially in dry environments or during long events, use a hydrating facial spray to refresh your makeup and add a burst of moisture to your skin.

By prioritizing hydration in your skincare and makeup routine, you create the ideal conditions for beautiful, glowing skin that enhances your makeup application and promotes overall skin health. This practice is especially important for black skin to maintain its natural radiance and prevent common issues like dryness and uneven texture.

Priming Your Skin for Makeup

Priming your skin before applying makeup is a critical step that can significantly enhance the appearance and longevity of your makeup. Primers work to create a smooth, flawless canvas, allowing foundation and other products to apply evenly and last longer. For black women, whose skin may exhibit unique characteristics such as increased oiliness or pronounced pores, using the right primer can make a dramatic difference in the overall look and wear of their makeup.

Benefits of Using a Primer

- **Smooths Skin Texture:** Primers can fill in pores, fine lines, and uneven textures, making the skin appear smoother.

- **Enhances Makeup Durability:** By forming a barrier between the skin and makeup, primers help prevent oils from breaking down makeup, thereby extending its wear.
- **Improves Color Payoff:** A good primer ensures that the true colors of your makeup come through, not dulled by the natural tone of your skin or absorbed unevenly.
- **Controls Shine:** Particularly for oily skin types, mattifying primers can keep the skin looking fresh and shine-free throughout the day.

Choosing the Right Primer

- **For Oily Skin:** Look for primers that are labeled as mattifying or oil-controlling to help reduce shine and oil breakthrough throughout the day.
- **For Dry Skin:** Hydrating primers or those with a creamy texture can add an extra layer of moisture, preventing makeup from clinging to dry patches.
- **For Combination Skin:** You might benefit from using different primers on different areas of your face, such as a mattifying primer on the T-zone and a hydrating primer on drier areas.
- **For Sensitive or Acne-Prone Skin:** Choose primers that are non-comedogenic and free from oils and fragrances to prevent irritation or breakouts.

Application Tips

- **Clean and Moisturize First:** Always start with clean, moisturized skin. Let your moisturizer absorb fully before applying primer to ensure it lays down smoothly.
- **Apply a Small Amount:** A little goes a long way with primer. Apply a small amount to your face using your fingertips, a brush, or a sponge. Focus on areas where your makeup tends to fade or where you have texture concerns.
- **Let it Settle:** Give your primer a minute or two to set before applying foundation. This allows the primer to create a seamless surface for makeup application.

Additional Considerations

- **Color-Correcting Primers:** If you have areas of hyperpigmentation, redness, or other color imbalances, consider using a color-correcting primer. Green primers can neutralize redness, while peach or orange primers are great for brightening dark spots common in black skin.
- **SPF Primers:** For an added layer of sun protection, opt for a primer with SPF. This is particularly important for black skin to prevent dark spots from getting darker and to maintain even skin tone.

By incorporating these priming strategies into your makeup routine, you ensure that your makeup not only looks flawless upon application but also maintains its beauty throughout the day. Primers are a secret weapon in achieving professional and long-lasting makeup looks, making them a must-have in the beauty arsenal of every black woman looking to perfect her makeup game.

Addressing Hyperpigmentation and Uneven Skin Tone

Hyperpigmentation and uneven skin tone are common concerns, especially for black women, due to the high melanin content in their skin which can make them more susceptible to visible marks following inflammation or irritation. Properly addressing these issues not only improves the appearance of your skin but also ensures a flawless makeup application.

Understanding Hyperpigmentation

Hyperpigmentation occurs when excess melanin is produced in certain areas of the skin, leading to dark spots or patches. This can result from various factors including sun exposure, hormonal changes, acne, and even injuries to the skin. Uneven skin tone can make skin appear patchy and can be challenging to cover with makeup.

Skincare Solutions

- **Sun Protection:** One of the most effective ways to prevent hyperpigmentation is to use sunscreen daily. UV rays can exacerbate dark spots, so applying a broad-spectrum SPF of at least 30 is crucial, even on cloudy days or indoors.
- **Topical Treatments:** Ingredients like vitamin C, hydroquinone, azelaic acid, niacinamide, and retinoids are known for their skin-lightening properties. These can help fade dark spots by inhibiting melanin production. Serums and creams containing these ingredients should be applied to clean skin before moisturizing.
- **Chemical Peels and Exfoliants:** Regular use of chemical exfoliants such as AHAs (glycolic acid, lactic acid) and BHAs (salicylic acid) can help accelerate cell turnover, removing the top layers of dead skin and diminishing the appearance of dark spots over time.

Makeup Techniques

- **Color Correctors:** Before applying foundation, use a color corrector to neutralize dark spots. Peach, orange, or red tinted correctors are effective for darker skin tones, as they can counteract the darkness and create an even base for foundation.
- **Buildable Foundation:** Opt for a foundation that offers buildable coverage. This allows you to increase coverage where you need it without applying a heavy layer over your entire face, maintaining a natural look.
- **Setting with Powder:** Use a translucent setting powder over areas where correctors and concealer are applied. This not only sets the makeup but also prevents it from shifting throughout the day and helps to even out the skin tone further.

Lifestyle Considerations

- **Healthy Diet:** A balanced diet rich in antioxidants can help protect the skin from damage that may lead to hyperpigmentation. Foods high in vitamins C and E are particularly beneficial.
- **Avoid Picking at the Skin:** Picking at acne, scabs, or other skin lesions can lead to scarring and dark spots. Keeping hands away from your face and treating breakouts with appropriate skincare products are crucial steps in preventing post-inflammatory hyperpigmentation.

Addressing hyperpigmentation and uneven skin tone requires a comprehensive approach that includes skincare, lifestyle adjustments, and specific makeup techniques. By integrating these strategies into your daily routine, you can achieve clearer, more radiant skin and enhance your overall makeup application. This not only boosts your confidence but also allows you to express your beauty without constraints.

Chapter 3: Makeup Basics for Beginners

Mastering the fundamentals of makeup application is essential for anyone beginning their beauty journey. This chapter focuses on the basics that every beginner should know, from selecting the perfect foundation shade to applying makeup for a flawless finish, and managing makeup on different skin types, particularly oily or dry skin.

Finding Your Perfect Shade

One of the most crucial aspects of makeup application, particularly for foundation and concealer, is finding your perfect shade. This ensures a seamless, natural look that enhances your skin without masking it. For black women, who often face challenges due to a broader range of skin tones and undertones, finding the right shade is especially important.

Understanding Undertones

- **Warm Undertones:** Skin has a golden, yellow, or peach hue. Look for foundations that have a yellow or golden base.
- **Cool Undertones:** Skin appears more bluish, pink, or red. Foundations with a pink or red base work best.
- **Neutral Undertones:** A mixture of both warm and cool hues, or your skin doesn't distinctly lean either way. Foundations that are neither overly yellow nor pink, often labeled as "neutral," are ideal.

Testing for the Right Shade

- **Swatch Test:** Apply a small amount of foundation along your jawline, not just on your hand. The right shade should blend invisibly into your skin without leaving visible lines.
- **Multiple Shades:** It's often beneficial to test multiple shades in a single session to see which one truly matches your skin tone. Apply side by side to compare.
- **Natural Light Check:** Always step outside or look in a window to see how the foundation looks in natural light. Artificial lighting can be misleading, as it may not accurately reflect the foundation's true color on your skin.

Tips for Finding Your Match

- **Ask for Samples:** Many stores provide samples, or you can purchase travel-sized versions to try out at home. This allows you to wear the foundation for a full day to see how it adapts to your natural skin oils and lighting changes.

- **Professional Help:** When in doubt, consult with a makeup professional at a beauty counter. They can provide guidance and often have a better eye for matching skin tones.
- **Custom Mixing:** Sometimes the best match comes from mixing two shades. If your skin tone changes with the seasons, you might also consider having a lighter shade for winter and a darker shade for summer, blending the two as needed.

Adjusting for Correct Coverage

- **Sheer to Full Coverage:** Depending on your preference and skin needs, the coverage level can also influence your shade choice. Sheer coverage can be more forgiving with slight shade mismatches, while full coverage requires a precise match to avoid looking unnatural.
- **Finish:** Consider the finish of the foundation—matte, dewy, or satin. Your skin type and the look you want to achieve can influence the best finish for you.

Finding the perfect shade is not just about matching your skin tone; it's about complementing your natural beauty and ensuring that your makeup enhances rather than conceals. This process might take some trial and error, but discovering your ideal foundation shade is a rewarding journey that elevates your makeup game to new heights.

Application Techniques for a Flawless Finish

Achieving a flawless makeup finish is not just about the products you use, but also how you apply them. This section provides detailed guidance on application techniques that can help you master the art of makeup and ensure a smooth, even, and lasting finish. These tips are particularly useful for beginners and are tailored to enhance the beauty of black skin.

Preparing the Skin

- **Start Clean:** Always begin with a clean face. Use a gentle cleanser that suits your skin type to remove any oils or impurities.
- **Moisturize:** Apply a moisturizer that matches your skin type. This helps to hydrate the skin and provides a smooth base for makeup application.
- **Prime:** Use a primer to create an even surface. This step is crucial for minimizing pores, smoothing fine lines, and helping makeup last longer.

Foundation Application

- **Tool Choice:** Use the right tool for your foundation type. For liquid foundations, a damp beauty sponge provides a dewy finish, while a brush can offer fuller coverage. Powders work best with a fluffy brush.
- **Technique:** Apply foundation starting from the center of the face and blend outward. This method ensures the most product remains where coverage is often needed most, preventing a heavy or cakey appearance around the edges of the face.
- **Build Gradually:** Layer your foundation gradually to achieve the desired coverage. This avoids a heavy makeup look and allows for more natural, breathable wear.

Concealer for Brightening and Coverage

- **Application:** Apply concealer under the eyes in a triangle shape to brighten the face and cover any dark circles. Also, dab concealer on spots or areas with hyperpigmentation. Choose a concealer one or two shades lighter than your foundation for brightening, or the exact match for spot treatment.
- **Blending:** Blend the edges thoroughly to integrate the concealer into your foundation seamlessly, using either a sponge, a brush, or your fingertips.

Setting Your Makeup

- **Translucent Powder:** Use a loose, translucent powder to set the makeup in key areas, like the under-eye, forehead, chin, and around the nose. This prevents creasing and controls shine.
- **Press and Roll Technique:** Use a powder puff or sponge to press and roll the powder onto the skin. This technique helps to set makeup without moving the product underneath.

Enhancing Features

- **Bronzer, Blush, and Highlighter:** Use these products to add depth and dimension. Apply bronzer to the perimeter of your face and beneath the cheekbones. Add blush to the apples of your cheeks for a healthy flush. Highlight the high points of your face, such as the cheekbones, brow bones, and cupid's bow, to enhance your natural glow.
- **Blend Well:** Ensure all products are blended thoroughly to avoid harsh lines. The goal is a seamless transition between colors and products.

- **Setting Spray:** Finish your makeup with a setting spray to lock everything in place and add an extra layer of hydration or mattification, depending on your skin type and desired finish.
- **Regular Check-ups:** Throughout the day, check and touch up your makeup if necessary. Blotting papers can help manage oil, and a compact powder is great for quick fixes.

By following these application techniques, you can achieve a makeup look that not only looks flawless but also feels comfortable and lasts all day. This foundation of skills is essential for any makeup enthusiast and will enhance your ability to present your best self to the world.

Dealing with Oily or Dry Skin Types

Understanding how to manage makeup application on different skin types is essential for achieving a flawless finish that lasts throughout the day. This section offers tailored advice for dealing with oily and dry skin types, which require specific approaches to ensure optimal makeup performance and appearance.

Oily Skin Management

Oily skin can pose challenges such as excess shine and makeup that seems to "slide off" or degrade throughout the day. Here are techniques to ensure makeup not only applies well but also stays put:

- **Priming:** Use an oil-free, mattifying primer to help control shine and create a smooth base. This type of primer minimizes the appearance of pores and helps to keep makeup in place.
- **Foundation:** Opt for oil-free, non-comedogenic foundations that offer a matte finish. These formulations help manage shine and prevent clogged pores.
- **Setting Powder:** After applying foundation, use a translucent setting powder to set your makeup. Apply the powder with a large fluffy brush or a powder puff to areas prone to oiliness, such as the T-zone.
- **Blotting Papers:** Keep blotting papers handy throughout the day to dab away excess oil without disturbing your makeup. This helps maintain a fresh look without adding more product.

- **Setting Spray:** Finish with a setting spray designed for oily skin. These sprays help to lock in makeup and control oil production for several hours.

Dry Skin Management

Dry skin can lead to makeup looking flaky, cakey, or uneven if not properly hydrated. Here's how to ensure a smooth and radiant finish:

- **Hydrating Primer:** Start with a hydrating primer to nourish the skin and smooth out any dry patches. This creates a pliable, moist base for further makeup application.
- **Moisture-Rich Foundation:** Choose foundations that are specifically designed for dry skin, preferably those with hydrating properties. Cream-based foundations are ideal as they provide moisture and coverage without settling into fine lines.
- **Gentle Application:** Apply foundation using a damp beauty sponge. This technique allows for a more hydrated application and avoids the abrasiveness of brushes, which can irritate dry skin and lift flaky patches.
- **Hydrating Setting Spray:** Instead of powder, which can dry out the skin further, use a hydrating setting spray to set your makeup. This can add a layer of moisture and keep your skin looking dewy and fresh.
- **Regular Exfoliation and Moisturization:** Incorporate exfoliation into your skincare routine to remove dead skin cells and allow moisturizers to penetrate more effectively. Always moisturize well at night and before makeup application.

By adapting your makeup routine to fit your specific skin type, whether oily or dry, you can enhance your overall makeup application and wear. These strategies are designed to address the unique challenges posed by each skin type, ensuring that your makeup looks its best from application to removal.

Chapter 4: Step-by-Step Makeup Tutorials

In this chapter, we delve into practical, step-by-step makeup tutorials tailored for black women, covering everything from a basic everyday look to more complex techniques for evening makeup and contouring. These tutorials are designed to help you master the art of makeup application for various occasions and needs.

Beginner Makeup Tutorial

1. Skin Preparation

- **Why It's Important**: Preparing your skin serves as the base for your makeup. It ensures your makeup applies smoothly and lasts longer. Starting with clean, hydrated skin can prevent makeup from looking patchy or cakey.
- **How to Do It**: Begin by cleansing your face to remove any dirt and oils. Apply a hydrating serum—such as one containing niacinamide which helps with skin hydration and adding glow. Follow up with a moisturizer or a hydrating primer that suits your skin type. Allow the moisturizer to absorb completely before proceeding to makeup application.

2. Foundation Application

- **Selecting the Right Foundation**: Choose a foundation that matches your skin type and undertone. For dry skin, opt for a hydrating, radiant foundation; for oily skin, look for a matte finish to help control shine.
- **Application Technique**: Dispense one pump of foundation onto the back of your hand. Using a foundation brush or a damp beauty sponge, start applying from the center of your face, blending outward. Focus on areas that need most coverage but avoid applying too much product immediately to prevent heavy, unnatural coverage.

3. Blending with Tools

- **Choosing Tools**: The choice between a beauty sponge and a brush depends on the desired finish and skin type. A damp beauty sponge is ideal for a dewy finish and works well with dry skin, as it helps in adding moisture. A kabuki brush is suitable for achieving a more polished, full-coverage finish.

- **Technique**: Use dabbing and rolling motions with a sponge to press the foundation into the skin for a seamless blend. With a brush, use circular, buffing motions to evenly distribute the product without streaking.

4. Concealer for Brightness

- **Purpose**: Concealer is used to cover imperfections such as dark circles, blemishes, and also to brighten areas of the face like under the eyes, the center of the forehead, and along the bridge of the nose.
- **Application**: Apply dots of concealer under the eyes, and on any spots or discoloration. Blend using the pointed end of a damp sponge or a concealer brush, ensuring the product melds into the skin without settling into lines.

5. Contouring Fundamentals

- **Why Contour**: Contouring helps define and sculpt the face, enhancing natural bone structure by mimicking shadows.
- **How to Contour**: Use a contour product two to three shades darker than your skin tone. Apply on the hollows of the cheeks, sides of the nose, jawline, and hairline. Blend using an angled contour brush, moving the product upwards to lift the face visually, avoiding harsh lines by blending thoroughly.

6. Setting the Base

- **Importance of Setting Powder**: Setting powder helps lock in the liquid and cream products, reducing creasing and extending wear.
- **Application**: Apply a translucent setting powder under the eyes and on other areas where you applied concealer to prevent the makeup from creasing. Use a larger fluffy brush to apply a setting powder matched to your skin tone over the rest of the face to blend everything smoothly.

7. Bronzer for Warmth

- **Choosing a Bronzer**: Select a bronzer with a warm tone to revive the complexion and add a healthy, sun-kissed glow.
- **Application Tips**: Apply the bronzer where the sun naturally hits the face—forehead, cheekbones, and along the jawline. Use a fluffy brush for a natural look, ensuring to blend the edges to avoid any obvious lines.

8. Blush Application

- **Effect of Blush**: Blush adds a natural flush of color, making your complexion look more vibrant and youthful.

- **How to Apply**: Smile to find the apples of your cheeks and apply the blush lightly, blending towards the hairline but concentrating the color on the cheeks. This enhances your face's natural contours without overwhelming your features.

9. Eyebrows and Eyelids

- **Eyebrows**: Shape and fill in your eyebrows with a brow pencil or mascara that matches your hair color. Use light strokes to keep the look natural, and brush through with a spoolie to distribute the color evenly.
- **Eyelids**: Apply a light layer of concealer on the eyelids to even out the skin tone. Set with a light powder before applying a neutral shade like a bronzer in the crease to define the eyes subtly.

10. Mascara and Lashes

- **Applying Mascara**: Wiggle the mascara wand at the base of your lashes and pull through to the tips to coat each lash thoroughly. This technique helps add volume and length.
- **Lashes**: For beginners, applying false lashes can be optional. If choosing to use them, select a natural-style lash and practice applying with a good adhesive.

11. Lips

- **Lining Lips**: Outline your lips with a lip liner slightly darker than your lipstick. This defines the shape and prevents color from bleeding.
- **Applying Lipstick**: Fill in your lips with a lipstick or gloss, starting from the center and blending outwards for a smooth finish.

12. Setting the Makeup

- **Final Touch**: Use a setting spray to help your makeup last longer and to meld the powders with the creams for a more natural, skin-like finish. This is particularly important for dry skin to add hydration.

Essential Makeup Techniques for a Flawless Look

Step 1: Primer Application

Purpose of Primer: Primer serves as the foundational base for all your makeup. Its primary role is to create a smooth, even surface on the skin, enhancing the application and longevity of the makeup that follows. A good primer not only improves the adherence of foundation and concealer but also helps minimize the appearance of pores, fine lines, and other skin imperfections.

Choosing the Right Primer: Selecting the right primer is crucial and should be based on your specific skin type and needs:

- **For Oily Skin**: Look for a matte primer that helps control excess oil and reduce shine throughout the day. A matte primer will typically contain ingredients like silica or silicone, which absorb oil and keep the skin looking smooth and matte. Example: e.l.f. Poreless Putty Primer.
- **For Dry Skin**: Choose a hydrating primer that contains moisturizing ingredients like hyaluronic acid or glycerin. These ingredients help to lock in moisture, keeping the skin hydrated and preventing makeup from clinging to dry patches. Example: Milani Supercharged Dew Primer.
- **For Combination Skin**: You might need to use two different primers for different areas of your face (a technique known as "primer cocktailing"). Use a mattifying primer in the T-zone to control oil and a hydrating primer on the cheeks and other dry areas.
- **For Long-Lasting Wear**: If longevity is your goal, especially in humid conditions or during long events, consider a gripping primer. These primers have a slightly tacky feel that helps makeup stick and stay put for hours. Example: e.l.f. Power Grip Primer.

Application Techniques: How you apply primer can make a significant difference in how your makeup looks and lasts:

1. **Clean and Moisturize**: Always start with a clean face. Apply your regular moisturizer and let it absorb fully into the skin before applying primer. This ensures that your skin is well-hydrated and that the primer can perform effectively.

2. **Apply a Small Amount**: You only need a pea-sized amount of primer for the entire face. Using too much can cause the primer to pill or interfere with the application of your foundation.
3. **Warm It Up**: Rub the primer between your fingers to warm it up before applying; this can make it easier to spread and blend into the skin.
4. **Focus on Problem Areas**: Pay special attention to areas where makeup tends to break down quickly, such as the T-zone, or where pores are more visible. Pat the primer into these areas instead of rubbing it to fill in pores and fine lines more effectively.
5. **Let It Set**: After applying the primer, give it a minute or two to set before moving on to foundation. This allows the primer to create a proper barrier between your skin and the makeup.

Testing Primers: Because everyone's skin is unique, what works for one person may not work for another. It's often a good idea to sample a primer to see how it interacts with your skin and your usual foundation. Many stores offer samples, or you can purchase travel-sized versions of products to test them out.

By following these steps and choosing the right product for your skin type, you can ensure that your makeup application starts off on the right foot, leading to a more flawless and lasting finish.

Step 2: Foundation Application

Purpose of Foundation: Foundation serves as the canvas for your makeup. Its primary function is to even out skin tone, cover imperfections, and provide a smooth, consistent surface for other makeup products. It can also offer various levels of coverage, from sheer to full, depending on the product and application technique used.

Choosing the Right Foundation: Selecting the ideal foundation involves understanding your skin's needs and preferences:

- **Skin Type Considerations**:
    - **Oily Skin**: Opt for oil-free, matte-finish foundations that help control shine and manage sebum production.
    - **Dry Skin**: Look for hydrating or dewy finish foundations that contain moisturizing ingredients to help keep the skin hydrated.
    - **Combination Skin**: You may need a balance between matte and hydrating foundations or apply different types depending on the face area.

-     o **Sensitive Skin**: Seek out hypoallergenic and fragrance-free formulas to reduce the risk of irritation.
- **Shade Matching**:
  - o **Match Your Undertone**: Determine if your undertone is cool, warm, or neutral. Cool undertones look best with foundations that have a pink or blue base, warm undertones with a yellow or golden base, and neutral undertones can look for a balance between the two.
  - o **Test in Natural Light**: Swatch foundations along your jawline, and check the color in natural light for the best match to ensure it blends seamlessly with your neck and chest.
- **Coverage Needs**:
  - o **Light Coverage**: Ideal for relatively clear skin or for those who prefer a natural look.
  - o **Medium Coverage**: Good for covering mild blemishes or uneven skin tone.
  - o **Full Coverage**: Best for covering more prominent imperfections or for those seeking a flawless finish.

Application Techniques: How you apply foundation can significantly affect its appearance and longevity:

1. **Preparation**: Begin with a well-moisturized and primed skin to ensure a smooth application. Allow the primer to fully set before applying foundation.
2. **Tools**:
   - o **Beauty Sponge**: Use damp for a sheer, dewy finish. Bounce the sponge over your skin to blend the foundation seamlessly.
   - o **Foundation Brush**: Use for more precise application and fuller coverage. Brushes with dense bristles give more coverage while stippling brushes offer a more airbrushed effect.
   - o **Fingers**: Suitable for those who want quick and light coverage. Warmth from your fingers can help melt the foundation into the skin, making it easier to blend.
3. **Application**:
   - o **Start at the Center**: Begin application in the center of the face where most people require more coverage and blend outward towards the hairline and jaw.
   - o **Build Coverage Gradually**: Apply foundation in thin layers and build up only in areas that need extra coverage to avoid a cakey look.
   - o **Blending**: Ensure there are no visible lines at the edges of your face, especially along the jawline and hairline.

4. **Setting**: Once your foundation is applied, set it with a suitable powder if necessary to increase its wear time and reduce shine in oily areas.

Additional Tips:

- **Hydration**: Even if you have oily skin, don't skip moisturizer. A hydrated skin will prevent the foundation from looking flaky.
- **Longevity**: For extended wear, consider using a setting spray after all your makeup is applied to lock everything in place.

By following these detailed steps and choosing the appropriate products, you can achieve a flawless foundation application that enhances your natural beauty and lasts throughout the day.

Step 3: Concealer Application

Purpose of Concealer: Concealer is a versatile product used to camouflage imperfections, brighten under-eye areas, and highlight specific features. It helps create a flawless complexion by covering dark circles, blemishes, redness, and uneven skin tone.

Choosing the Right Concealer: Selecting the perfect concealer involves considering various factors:

- **Coverage Level**:
    - **Full Coverage**: Ideal for concealing intense discolorations or prominent blemishes.
    - **Medium Coverage**: Suitable for everyday use to cover minor imperfections without feeling heavy.
    - **Sheer Coverage**: Best for highlighting and brightening the under-eye area without adding additional coverage.
- **Formulation**:
    - **Liquid Concealer**: Offers blendability and versatility, suitable for most skin types.
    - **Cream Concealer**: Provides more coverage and is ideal for drier skin types.
    - **Stick Concealer**: Convenient for spot-concealing and provides buildable coverage.
- **Undertone**:
    - **Peach/Salmon**: Great for neutralizing dark circles and blue-toned imperfections.

- ○ **Yellow**: Helps counteract redness and brighten the skin.
- ○ **Neutral**: Matches the skin tone without adding warmth or coolness.

Application Techniques: Mastering the application of concealer can significantly enhance your overall makeup look:

1. **Preparation**: Start with a clean, moisturized face. Apply primer if desired to create a smooth base for concealer application.
2. **Tools**:
   - ○ **Concealer Brush**: Offers precision and control, ideal for spot-concealing blemishes or applying concealer to targeted areas.
   - ○ **Beauty Sponge**: Provides a seamless, airbrushed finish. Dampen the sponge before use to blend concealer effortlessly.
   - ○ **Fingers**: Warm up the product by gently tapping it onto the skin, then blend using a patting motion.
3. **Application**:
   - ○ **Under Eyes**: Apply concealer in a triangular shape beneath the eyes, extending towards the temples. This technique brightens the entire eye area and conceals dark circles.
   - ○ **Blemishes/Imperfections**: Dab concealer directly onto the affected area using a precise brush or fingertip. Blend the edges seamlessly into the surrounding skin for a natural finish.
   - ○ **Highlighting**: Apply concealer to the high points of the face, such as the bridge of the nose, center of the forehead, cupid's bow, and chin, to add dimension and luminosity.
4. **Blending**:
   - ○ Blend concealer using gentle tapping or dabbing motions to ensure seamless integration with the foundation.
   - ○ Avoid harsh rubbing or dragging motions, especially around delicate areas like the under-eye area, to prevent creasing or cakeiness.
5. **Setting**:
   - ○ To prolong the wear of your concealer and prevent creasing, set it with a translucent or color-matched setting powder using a fluffy brush or makeup sponge.

Additional Tips:

- • **Color Correction**: Use color-correcting concealers (e.g., green for redness, peach/salmon for dark circles) before applying regular concealer to target specific concerns.

- **Layering**: For stubborn blemishes or intense discoloration, layer concealer in thin, buildable layers rather than applying a thick coat all at once.

By following these comprehensive steps and selecting the appropriate concealer and tools for your needs, you can achieve a flawless complexion with targeted coverage and a natural-looking finish.

Step 4: Foundation Application

Purpose of Foundation: Foundation serves as the base for your makeup, providing coverage, evening out skin tone, and creating a smooth canvas for further makeup application. It helps blur imperfections and enhances the skin's natural beauty.

Choosing the Right Foundation: Finding the perfect foundation involves considering several factors tailored to your skin type, tone, and preferences:

- **Coverage Level**:
    - **Sheer/Light Coverage**: Offers a natural, dewy finish and is suitable for everyday wear.
    - **Medium Coverage**: Provides a balance between natural and full coverage, ideal for evening out skin tone and concealing minor imperfections.
    - **Full Coverage**: Conceals blemishes, discoloration, and acne scars for a flawless complexion, often with a matte finish.
- **Finish**:
    - **Matte**: Absorbs excess oil and provides a shine-free, velvety finish, ideal for oily or combination skin.
    - **Dewy**: Adds luminosity and radiance to the skin, perfect for dry or dull complexions.
    - **Natural/Satin**: Strikes a balance between matte and dewy, offering a natural-looking finish suitable for most skin types.
- **Undertone**:
    - **Warm**: Has yellow or golden undertones, complementing peachy or olive skin tones.
    - **Cool**: Contains pink or blue undertones, suitable for fair skin with pink or blue undertones.
    - **Neutral**: Balances both warm and cool undertones, suitable for a wide range of skin tones.

Application Techniques: Mastering foundation application ensures a flawless base for the rest of your makeup:

1. **Preparation**: Begin with a clean, moisturized face. Apply primer if desired to extend the wear of your foundation and smooth out the skin's texture.
2. **Tools**:
    - **Foundation Brush**: Provides controlled application and allows for precise blending.
    - **Beauty Sponge**: Offers seamless blending and a natural finish, especially when dampened before use.
    - **Fingers**: Warm up the foundation by rubbing it between your fingertips, then gently pat and blend it onto the skin for a natural look.
3. **Application**:
    - **Start in the Center**: Apply foundation to the center of the face (forehead, nose, cheeks, and chin), where most coverage is needed, then blend outward towards the hairline and jawline.
    - **Build Coverage Gradually**: Begin with a small amount of product and gradually build up coverage as needed, focusing on areas with blemishes or discoloration.
    - **Blend Thoroughly**: Use tapping or stippling motions to blend foundation seamlessly into the skin, ensuring no harsh lines or uneven patches.
4. **Layering**:
    - If additional coverage is desired, apply a second layer of foundation only to areas that need extra coverage, such as blemishes or redness, to avoid a heavy, cakey look.
5. **Set the Foundation**:
    - To enhance longevity and prevent transfer, set the foundation with a light dusting of translucent or setting powder using a fluffy brush or makeup sponge.

Additional Tips:

- **Color Matching**: Test foundation shades on your jawline or neck to ensure a seamless blend with your natural skin tone.
- **Customization**: Mix different foundations or add illuminating drops to achieve your desired finish or coverage level.
- **Blend into the Hairline and Neck**: Ensure seamless blending by feathering the foundation into the hairline and down the neck to avoid a noticeable line of demarcation.

Step 5: Concealer and Setting Powder

Purpose of Concealer and Setting Powder: Concealer is used to cover imperfections such as dark circles, blemishes, and discolorations, enhancing the skin's appearance by creating a more even and flawless complexion. Setting powder helps to lock the concealer and foundation in place, reducing shine and providing a smooth, long-lasting finish.

Choosing the Right Concealer and Setting Powder: Selecting the right products depends on your skin's needs and the specific concerns you wish to address:

- **Concealer:**
  - **Coverage**: Choose a coverage level that matches your needs—full coverage for significant imperfections, medium for everyday use, and light for minor blemishes and brightening.
  - **Formula**: Consider the formula that works best for your skin type. Liquid concealers are versatile and suitable for most skin types, cream concealers offer dense coverage and are great for dry skin, while stick concealers are good for targeted application.
  - **Color Correcting**: Use color correctors (green to neutralize redness, peach/salmon to counteract blue or purple under-eye circles) before applying a skin-toned concealer.
- **Setting Powder:**
  - **Types**: Choose between loose and pressed powder based on your preference. Loose powders are ideal for a natural, lightweight finish, while pressed powders are better for touch-ups and more precise application.
  - **Finish**: Opt for a matte finish to reduce shine or a translucent setting powder to avoid altering the color of your foundation and concealer.

Application Techniques:

1. **Concealer Application:**
   - **Preparation**: Ensure your under-eye area is moisturized to prevent the concealer from caking.
   - **Tool Selection**: Use a concealer brush for precise application or a damp beauty sponge for a blended, airbrushed finish.
   - **Technique**: Apply concealer in a triangular shape under the eyes to brighten the entire area, and dab onto blemishes or redness. Blend by gently tapping to merge seamlessly with the foundation.
2. **Setting Powder Application:**

- Preparation: After applying concealer, allow it to set for a moment to avoid smudging.
  - **Tool Selection**: Use a fluffy brush for a light, airy application of loose powder, or a puff for pressed powder to press the powder into the skin.
  - **Technique**: Apply a small amount of powder to set the concealer. Focus on areas prone to creasing or oiliness, such as under the eyes, the T-zone, and over blemishes. Use a pressing motion rather than rubbing to avoid displacing the concealer.

Layering and Blending:

- **Layering**: If additional coverage is needed, apply layers of concealer sparingly to avoid buildup. Set each layer with a small amount of powder to maintain coverage and extend wear.
- **Blending**: Ensure all edges are blended into the surrounding skin and foundation to prevent visible lines. Use a clean brush or sponge to smooth out any excess product gently.

Final Checks and Adjustments:

- **Check Coverage and Creasing**: Examine your face in different lighting to ensure coverage is even and there are no creases. Adjust by blending out creases and adding more powder as needed.
- **Longevity**: For all-day wear, consider a final mist of setting spray to lock in the makeup and keep it looking fresh.

By following these detailed steps for applying concealer and setting powder, you can effectively conceal imperfections and ensure your makeup base remains flawless and durable throughout the day. This foundation of a well-prepared skin canvas is crucial for enhancing subsequent makeup application, whether for everyday wear or special occasions.

Step 6: Contouring and Bronzing

Purpose of Contouring and Bronzing: Contouring and bronzing are techniques used to define and enhance facial features. Contouring creates shadows to define and sculpt the face, while bronzing adds warmth and a sun-kissed glow, giving the skin a healthy, vibrant appearance.

Choosing the Right Products: Selecting appropriate contour and bronzer products depends on your skin tone and the effect you wish to achieve:

- **Contour Products**:
  - **Shade**: Choose a contour shade that is two to three shades darker than your natural skin tone with a matte finish to mimic natural shadows.
  - **Type**: Powders are easier for beginners to control and blend, while creams offer a more dramatic, defined look.
- **Bronzer**:
  - **Shade**: Opt for a bronzer that is warm-toned but not too orange. It should enhance your skin tone without overpowering it.
  - **Type**: Powder bronzers are recommended for beginners for ease of application and blending.

Application Techniques:

1. **Contour Application**:
   - **Tools**: Use an angled contour brush for precise application or a fluffy brush for a softer, more diffused look.
   - **Technique**:
     - Identify the natural shadows of your face, typically under the cheekbones, along the hairline, jawline, and sides of the nose.
     - Apply the contour product in a line along these areas.
     - Blend upwards or towards the hairline for the cheekbones and downwards for the jawline to create a natural shadow effect.
     - For the nose, use a smaller brush to lightly draw lines down from the bridge to the tip and blend thoroughly.
2. **Bronzer Application**:
   - **Tools**: Use a fluffy brush that can disperse the product evenly.
   - **Technique**:
     - Swipe the bronzer where the sun naturally hits your face: the top of the forehead, cheekbones, and along the jawline.
     - Apply in a "3" shape on the sides of the face, blending from the forehead, below the cheekbones, and down to the jawline.
     - Use circular motions to blend the bronzer into the skin for a natural, sun-kissed effect.
     - Avoid applying too much product at once; build it up gradually to achieve the desired intensity.

Blending and Layering:

- **Blending**: Ensure that both the contour and bronzer are well blended to avoid harsh lines. This can be achieved by using a clean brush or a beauty sponge to soften the edges.

- **Layering**: If needed, layer the bronzer over the contour for additional warmth, especially on the cheekbones and the periphery of the face.

Final Adjustments:

- **Check Boundaries**: Ensure there are no distinct lines between your contour, bronzer, and foundation. Everything should seamlessly blend into each other.
- **Adjust Intensity**: If you've applied too much, you can tone it down by going over it with a bit of foundation or setting powder.
- **Highlight**: To complete the sculpting, apply a highlighter to the high points of the face (cheekbones, bridge of the nose, cupid's bow) to create contrast and enhance the effect of the contour and bronzer.

By mastering these techniques and choosing the right products, you can effectively sculpt, define, and enhance your facial features, adding dimension and warmth to your makeup look. This step is crucial for achieving a balanced and polished overall appearance.

Step 7: Blush Application

Purpose of Blush: Blush is used to add a healthy, natural flush of color to the cheeks, enhancing the complexion and bringing life and vibrancy to the face. It helps create a more youthful appearance and can balance the effects of contouring and bronzing by adding warmth and dimension.

Choosing the Right Blush: Selecting the appropriate blush involves considering your skin tone, the finish you desire, and the overall look you want to achieve:

- **Color Choice**:
    - For cool undertones, shades like pink or light rose enhance the natural flush.
    - For warm undertones, peach, coral, or earthy tones work best to complement the skin.
    - For neutral undertones, almost any color can work, but muted versions of peach or pink are particularly flattering.
- **Formula**:
    - **Powder Blush**: Ideal for oily to combination skin, easy to apply, and great for beginners.
    - **Cream Blush**: Best for dry or mature skin, offering a dewy finish.
    - **Liquid Blush**: Provides a natural, stain-like effect, suitable for all skin types and especially beneficial for achieving a layered, long-lasting color.

Application Techniques:

1. **Tool Selection**:
    - **For Powder Blush**: Use a soft, fluffy brush that can diffuse color softly on the cheeks.
    - **For Cream Blush**: Fingers or a sponge work well for blending out edges seamlessly.
    - **For Liquid Blush**: A stippling brush or fingers for placement and blending, ensuring a more controlled and even application.
2. **Application Process**:
    - **Smile and Apply**: Smile to find the apples of your cheeks. Begin application on the apples and blend upwards towards the temples and back towards the earlobes to create a lifted effect.
    - **Intensity Control**: Start with a light hand, picking up a small amount of product. Build intensity gradually to avoid over-application. Tap off excess blush from the brush to ensure a light application.
    - **Blending**: Blend thoroughly to diffuse edges, making the blush look like a natural part of your skin rather than sitting on top.
3. **Layering and Adjusting**:
    - **Layering**: If using cream or liquid blush, apply before powder products to prevent them from caking. For powder blush, apply after foundation and powder setting.
    - **Adjusting Color**: If you've applied too much, go over the area with a clean brush dipped in a little foundation powder to mute the intensity.
    - **Harmonizing with Makeup**: Ensure the blush color harmonizes with the overall makeup look, including eyeshadow and lip color, to create a cohesive appearance.

Final Checks:

- **Natural Lighting Check**: After applying, check your makeup in natural light to ensure it appears as desired and adjust accordingly.
- **Longevity Enhancement**: Set cream or liquid blushes with a light dusting of translucent powder to enhance their longevity if needed, especially for oily skin types.

By following these detailed steps and selecting the appropriate blush and tools for your needs, you can achieve a naturally flushed, vibrant look that enhances your facial features and complements your overall makeup. Blush is essential for adding life back to the complexion after the application of foundation and contouring products.

Step 8: Finishing Touches

Purpose of Finishing Touches: The final steps in a makeup routine—applying setting spray, lip liner, lipstick, and potentially eyeshadow—are crucial for achieving a polished, cohesive look that enhances your features and ensures the longevity of your makeup.

Setting Spray:

- **Purpose**: Locks makeup in place, melds the layers together for a more seamless finish, and can either mattify or add a dewy glow depending on the formula.
- **Application**:
    - Hold the spray at arm's length and mist your face in an "X" and "T" pattern to cover all areas evenly.
    - Allow the spray to dry naturally to set the makeup, providing a lasting finish that reduces smudging, fading, and creasing throughout the day.

Lip Liner and Lipstick:

- **Purpose**: Defines the lips, prevents lipstick from feathering, and enhances the fullness of your lips.
- **Lip Liner**:
    - Choose a shade that closely matches your lipstick or a neutral shade that matches your natural lip color for versatility.
    - Outline the natural border of your lips to define their shape, and if desired, slightly overline to create the illusion of fuller lips.
    - Fill in the lips lightly with liner before applying lipstick to increase the longevity and intensity of the color.
- **Lipstick**:
    - Apply your chosen shade, starting from the center of the lips and working outward.
    - Blot and reapply if necessary to build up lasting coverage and depth of color.
    - For a precise application, use a lip brush, especially for bold or dark colors.

Eyeshadow Application (if applicable):

- **Purpose**: Enhances the eyes and complements the overall makeup look.
- **Basic Application**:
    - Start with an eyeshadow primer to ensure longevity and vibrant color payoff.
    - Apply a neutral base color all over the lid to set the primer.
    - Use a slightly darker shade in the crease to define the eye shape, blending thoroughly to avoid harsh lines.
    - Apply a lighter, shimmer shade to the inner corners and brow bone to highlight and open up the eyes.
    - Blend all shades together seamlessly for a polished look.

Final Review and Adjustments:

- **Review**: Examine your makeup in different lighting to ensure everything is blended smoothly and looks balanced.
- **Adjustments**: Use a clean brush or sponge to blend or remove excess product, particularly around the eyes and lips.
- **Hydration**: If the skin looks too matte or powdery, a hydrating mist can refresh the makeup and add a natural glow.

Additional Tips:

- **Eyeshadow for Beginners**: Stick to a simple palette with neutral shades for easy blending and a versatile look.
- **Lip Enhancements**: For extra volume, apply a gloss over your lipstick, focusing on the center of the lips.
- **Setting Mist for Skincare**: If you have dry skin, look for setting sprays with hydrating ingredients like hyaluronic acid or glycerin to keep the skin moisturized and make the makeup look more dewy.

By meticulously applying these finishing touches, you can ensure your makeup not only looks stunning but also holds up beautifully throughout your activities. These steps encapsulate all the techniques needed to finalize your makeup application, enhancing durability, and overall aesthetic appeal.

Basic Everyday Look

An everyday makeup look should enhance your natural beauty, providing a fresh and polished appearance without too much complexity. This tutorial focuses on creating a simple yet effective daily look that is perfect for work, school, or casual outings, specifically tailored for black women.

1. Skin Prep

- **Cleanse and Moisturize:** Start with a clean face and apply a moisturizer that suits your skin type to ensure your makeup goes on smoothly.
- **Prime:** Use a light primer to help makeup last longer and to create a smooth canvas. If you have oily skin, consider a mattifying primer; if you have dry skin, opt for a hydrating one.

2. Foundation

- **Application:** Apply a lightweight foundation or a tinted moisturizer for a more natural look. Use a beauty sponge or a foundation brush to blend the product evenly across your face, making sure to match your skin tone perfectly for a seamless effect.
- **Blend:** Ensure there are no visible lines at the edges, especially along your jawline and hairline.

3. Concealer

- **Under Eyes:** Apply a concealer under your eyes to brighten the area. Choose a shade that is slightly lighter than your foundation.
- **Blemishes:** Dab a small amount of concealer on any blemishes or dark spots. Use a shade that matches your foundation to blend it seamlessly.

4. Setting Powder

- **Light Dusting:** Use a translucent setting powder to set the areas where you applied concealer and any other oily areas. This step helps prevent creasing and ensures your base makeup stays intact throughout the day.

5. Blush

- **Natural Flush:** Choose a blush that complements your skin tone. Peach or coral shades look beautiful on darker skin. Apply lightly to the apples of your cheeks to bring a healthy color to your face.

6. Eyebrows

- **Fill and Shape:** Use an eyebrow pencil or powder close to your hair color to fill in sparse areas. Shape your eyebrows to frame your face, focusing on a natural look.

7. Eyelashes

- **Mascara:** Apply a coat of mascara to curl and define your lashes, opening up your eyes. If you prefer, use an eyelash curler before applying mascara for extra lift.

8. Lips

- **Natural Lip Color:** Finish your look with a tinted lip balm or a gloss for a soft, natural lip. Choose a color that enhances your natural lip color and adds a bit of shine.

9. Setting Spray

- **Hydrate and Set:** Mist your face with a setting spray to keep everything in place and to add a bit of hydration for a dewy finish.

This basic everyday look is designed to be quick and easy, enhancing your natural beauty without appearing overdone. It's perfect for those new to makeup or those who prefer a minimalist approach but still want to look put-together every day.

Transitioning to a Nighttime Look

Elevating your makeup from a day to a night look allows you to experiment with more dramatic and bold choices, perfect for evenings out, dinners, or special occasions. This tutorial will guide you on how to effortlessly transition your basic everyday makeup into a glamorous nighttime look, specifically tailored for black women.

1. Enhance the Foundation

- **Build Coverage:** If your daytime foundation is light, apply a little more foundation or a concealer to areas that need more coverage for a flawless evening look. Blend well for a seamless finish.
- **Matte Finish:** For oily skin, touch up with a mattifying powder to control shine, especially in the T-zone area.

2. Intensify the Eyes

- **Darker Eyeshadows:** Switch from neutral to darker shades like deep browns, golds, or even metallics to add depth and drama. Apply a darker shadow in the crease and outer corners of your eyes.
- **Eyeliner:** Apply a black or dark brown eyeliner along the top lash line. Consider extending it slightly for a winged effect, which adds an element of sophistication.
- **Smudge:** Use a smudge brush to softly blend a dark eyeshadow or eyeliner under your lower lashes for a smoky effect.

3. Lashes

- **False Lashes:** For an extra glamorous touch, apply false eyelashes. Choose fuller, longer lashes for an eye-catching look.
- **Extra Mascara:** If you opt not to use false lashes, apply an additional coat of volumizing mascara to both top and bottom lashes to make your eyes pop.

4. Highlight and Contour

- **Contour:** Reinforce your contouring to define your facial features more dramatically under evening lighting. Use a contour powder or cream beneath your cheekbones, along your jawline, and at the temples.
- **Highlight:** Apply a highlighter more generously on the high points of your face like cheekbones, down the bridge of your nose, and the cupid's bow to enhance your features and add a radiant glow.

5. Bolder Blush

- **Deeper Shade:** Opt for a slightly deeper shade of blush to complement the stronger eye and lip makeup. Apply it on the apples of the cheeks and blend upwards towards the temples.

6. Statement Lips

- **Bold Color:** Switch your day lip color to a bolder shade like red, deep berry, or plum. For a precise application, line your lips with a matching lip liner before applying lipstick.
- **Matte or Glossy:** Depending on your preference, choose a matte lipstick for a sophisticated look or a glossy finish for added glamour.

7. Set Your Makeup

- **Setting Spray:** Finish with a long-lasting setting spray to ensure your makeup stays put throughout the night.

With these steps, you can easily transform your makeup from a subtle daytime appearance to a more dramatic and elegant evening look. This transition allows you to play with colors and intensities that you might normally reserve for special occasions, perfectly suiting the nighttime vibe.

Top 10 Makeup Mistakes to Avoid

1. Skipping Moisturizer: One of the biggest makeup blunders is skipping moisturizer, especially if you don't consider your skin type. Using the right moisturizer forms a smooth canvas and ensures that your makeup doesn't look patchy or dry.

2. Not Letting Moisturizer Absorb: Always wait at least five minutes after applying your moisturizer before starting your makeup. This allows your skin to fully absorb the moisturizer, preventing it from mixing with your foundation which can affect the makeup's durability and appearance.

3. Using the Wrong Moisturizer: Choosing a moisturizer that isn't suited for your skin type can lead to issues like excess oiliness or dry patches. For oily skin, opt for an oil-free, water-based moisturizer; for dry skin, a deeply hydrating moisturizer works best.

4. Foundation Misapplication: Avoid applying foundation immediately after your moisturizer or using the wrong shade. Ensure that the foundation matches your skin tone by testing it on your face or chest, rather than your neck, which might have a different shade.

5. Neglecting Tools Hygiene: Using makeup brushes or sponges that are not clean can lead to uneven application and skin breakouts. Always use clean, fresh applicators to keep your makeup smooth and your skin healthy.

6. Incorrect Concealer Use: Selecting the wrong type of concealer can make under-eye creases more prominent. Opt for a liquid concealer for a more natural, crease-less finish under the eyes, and remember to let it sit for a few minutes before blending.

7. Overusing Setting Powder: Applying too much setting powder, especially under the eyes, can lead to a dry, cakey appearance. Use just enough to set your makeup and ensure it's well-blended to avoid a heavy look.

8. Improper Contour Placement: Contour should mimic natural shadows, so avoid applying it too heavily or in the wrong places. Use a light hand and blend well to achieve a naturally sculpted look.

9. Choosing the Wrong Highlighter: Avoid highlighters that look too powdery or sit heavily on your skin. Aim for products that offer a subtle glow to enhance your features without overwhelming them.

10. Neglecting Setting Spray: A good setting spray is essential to lock your makeup in place and prevent it from moving throughout the day. Choose a setting spray that complements your skin type—hydrating mists for dry skin and mattifying formulas for oily skin.

By steering clear of these common makeup mistakes, you can achieve a more flawless and lasting makeup look. Remember, the key to perfect makeup lies not only in the products you choose but also in how you apply them.

Step-by-Step Makeup Tutorial for Hot and Humid Weather

Step 1: Prepare Your Skin

- **Moisturize**: Start by cleansing your face to remove any impurities. Apply a moisturizer that's suitable for your skin type. For all skin types, especially in humid conditions, an oil-free moisturizer like Neutrogena Hydro Boost Water Gel is recommended. For a more plumping effect, try Bobbi Brown Vitamin Enriched Face Base, which is also oil-free and hydrating.

Step 2: Apply Primer

- **Why It's Important**: A primer not only provides a smooth base for makeup application but also protects your skin from the chemicals in makeup, preventing clogged pores and breakouts.
- **Product Recommendations**: Use a primer that has silica or silicone for its oil-absorbing properties. For dry skin, Cover FX Mattifying Booster Drops or NYX Hydra Touch Primer works well. For oily skin or skin with visible pores, try NYX Pore Filler Primer.

Step 3: Set the Base with Translucent Powder

- **Choice of Powder**: Avoid pressed powders or powder foundations as they add too much coverage, which can clog pores and increase sweat production. Instead, use a translucent setting powder that matches your skin tone.

- **Application Technique**: Use a makeup sponge to press the translucent powder onto the skin, focusing on areas prone to oiliness such as the T-zone. Recommended products include Laura Mercier Translucent Setting Powder in Medium Deep or Milani Make It Last Setting Powder in Medium to Deep.

Step 4: Apply Setting Spray

- **Purpose**: A setting spray helps to lock in the base layers (primer and powder) and prevents makeup from moving or melting off.
- **How to Use**: After applying the powder, generously mist your face with a setting spray that has long-lasting properties. Urban Decay All Nighter Setting Spray is great for up to 12 hours of wear. For dry skin, Milani Make It Last Dewy Setting Spray is an affordable option.
- **Drying Time**: Allow the setting spray to dry for about two minutes before proceeding with foundation application. This helps to seal the base and prevents oils from breaking through.

Step 5: Foundation Application

- **Moderation is Key**: Apply just one pump of foundation at a time to build up coverage without suffocating the skin. Start with areas that are less prone to sweating, like the cheeks and forehead.
- **Technique**: Use the remaining product on the applicator to lightly cover areas that tend to sweat more, such as the nose and cupid's bow. This approach helps minimize the amount of product in sweat-prone areas, reducing the risk of makeup separation.

Step 6: Touch-ups Throughout the Day

- **Using Blotting Powder**: If oils appear later in the day, opt for blotting powder rather than adding more pressed powder. Blotting powder, like white translucent powder, helps remove oil without adding coverage, maintaining a natural look.
- **Alternative**: Blotting papers are also effective for removing excess oil and sweat without disturbing your makeup.

Final Note: Proper skin preparation and strategic product application are key to maintaining a flawless look in hot and humid weather. Be sure to adapt the products and techniques to suit your specific skin type and environmental conditions.

Special Techniques for Contouring and Highlighting

Contouring and highlighting are powerful makeup techniques that can sculpt, define, and enhance your facial features, creating a more structured and radiant look. This tutorial will focus on how to effectively use these techniques, especially for black women, to highlight their natural beauty and define their features with precision.

1. Understanding Contouring and Highlighting

- **Contouring:** This technique involves using a matte product that is two shades darker than your skin tone to create shadows and define areas such as the cheeks, jawline, and temples.
- **Highlighting:** Highlighting uses light-reflecting products to draw attention to the high points of the face, such as the cheekbones, brow bones, bridge of the nose, and cupid's bow.

2. Selecting the Right Products

- **Contour Products:** Choose a contour product (powder, cream, or stick) that complements your undertone. For deeper skin tones, products with a cool to neutral undertone can often look more natural.
- **Highlight Products:** Select a highlighter that suits your skin tone; golden or bronze tones often work beautifully on black skin, providing a warm, radiant glow.

3. Technique for Contouring

- **Map Out Your Face:** Use the contour product to trace the areas you want to define. For cheekbones, make a line starting from your ear towards the corner of your mouth, stopping midway. For the jawline, apply along the jaw to enhance its natural line. Contour the sides of your nose to slim and define it.
- **Blending:** Use a contour brush or damp beauty sponge to blend the product into your skin. Ensure there are no harsh lines; blending is key to a natural-looking contour.

4. Technique for Highlighting

- **Application Areas:** Apply your highlighter to the tops of your cheekbones, down the bridge of your nose, on the brow bone, above the cupid's bow, and a tiny bit on the chin.

- **Blend Softly:** Using a fluffy brush or your fingertips, blend the highlighter well into your skin. The goal is to create a subtle glow that enhances your features without looking too shiny.

5. Integrating Both Techniques

- **Layering:** After contouring, apply your foundation and concealer as usual, then proceed to highlight. This helps integrate all the products seamlessly for a cohesive look.
- **Setting:** To ensure longevity and to prevent the contour and highlight from shifting, lightly dust setting powder over your face. Use a setting spray for an added layer of security and a fresh finish.

6. Adjustments and Precision

- **Tailor to Your Face Shape:** Adjust the placement and intensity of both contour and highlight according to your specific face shape. Different face shapes benefit from different techniques (e.g., contouring under the cheekbones is great for round faces, while highlighting above the cheekbones suits heart-shaped faces).
- **Use the Right Tools:** For contouring, angled brushes or sticks are ideal for precise application. For highlighting, a fan brush or a smaller, fluffy brush works best for a controlled and targeted application.

By mastering these special techniques for contouring and highlighting, you can transform your makeup look, enhancing your natural beauty with depth and dimension. Whether for daily wear or special occasions, these skills allow you to confidently accentuate your best features.

Applying Eye Makeup for Different Occasions

Eye makeup can dramatically alter your look, making it an essential skill to master for any occasion. This tutorial will guide you through various eye makeup styles suitable for different events, ensuring that you can confidently enhance your eyes to match your overall look and the setting.

1. Casual Day Look

For everyday activities like going to work or running errands, a simple and understated eye makeup look is ideal.

- **Neutral Shadows:** Start with a light, neutral eyeshadow across your entire eyelid to even out the skin tone.
- **Soft Definition:** Use a medium brown or taupe shade in the crease of your eye to add depth. Blend well to avoid any harsh lines.
- **Mascara:** Apply one to two coats of mascara to open up the eyes and keep the look fresh and simple.
- **Optional Liner:** For a bit more definition without going too bold, apply a thin line of brown eyeliner along the upper lash line.

2. Professional Settings

For work meetings or professional events, keeping your eye makeup polished and subtle is key.

- **Matte Shades:** Use matte eyeshadows as they are less distracting and more suitable for professional environments. Stick with neutral colors.
- **Enhanced Definition:** Apply a darker shade in the outer corner and blend into the crease to subtly enhance eye shape.
- **Clean Eyeliner:** Use a gel or liquid eyeliner to draw a precise line along the top lash line. A small wing at the end can elevate the look without being too dramatic.
- **Neutral Mascara:** Finish with black mascara, focusing on the roots to avoid clumpy lashes.

3. Evening Events

Evening events or parties are the perfect occasion to experiment with more dramatic and bold eye makeup.

- **Darker Shadows:** Opt for deeper or vibrant eyeshadow colors like plums, deep greens, or shimmering golds. Apply a darker color in the crease and outer V of the eye to create a smoky effect.
- **Glitter or Metallics:** Add a touch of glamour with a shimmering or metallic shadow on the center of the lid. This catches the light beautifully, especially in low-light settings.
- **Bold Eyeliner:** Consider a bold winged eyeliner or even colored eyeliner to make a statement. Black liquid eyeliner can provide a dramatic and polished look.
- **False Lashes:** For added drama, apply a pair of false lashes that complement the shape of your eyes, enhancing both the length and volume.

4. Special Occasions

For weddings, galas, or other special events where you want to look your best, combining elegance with drama is key.

- **Elegant Smoky Eye:** Create a classic smoky eye with layers of shadow, starting with a light base, a medium hue in the crease, and a dark color at the outer corners and along the lash lines.
- **Highlight Inner Corners:** Use a light, shimmery eyeshadow or a highlighter in the inner corners of your eyes to brighten and open up the eye area.
- **Defined Lashes:** Multiple coats of volumizing mascara or a set of dramatic false eyelashes can finalize the look, ensuring your eyes are the focal point.
- **Blend Everything Well:** Ensure all eyeshadows are blended seamlessly. Harsh lines can detract from the sophistication of your look.

By mastering these different styles and techniques for eye makeup, you can ensure that your eyes always complement your outfit and the occasion. Whether keeping it simple for day-to-day activities or going bold for a night out, these tips will help you enhance your natural eye shape and color beautifully.

Chapter 5: Foundation and Concealer

Mastering the application of foundation and concealer is essential for creating a flawless makeup base. This chapter provides a detailed guide on how to apply these products effectively, along with tips to ensure they offer long-lasting coverage, particularly beneficial for black women whose skin may have unique concerns such as oil control and hyperpigmentation.

Detailed Guide on Application

Achieving a flawless makeup base is foundational to any great look. This guide provides detailed steps for applying foundation and concealer, tailored to enhance the natural beauty of black women's skin, which often requires specific considerations for even and long-lasting coverage.

Foundation Application

Applying foundation effectively is key to achieving a flawless makeup look. For black women, it's particularly important to choose the right shade and formula to enhance the natural beauty of their skin tone and texture. Here is a detailed guide on how to apply foundation for a smooth, even finish.

1. Preparation:

- **Cleanse:** Start with a clean face to ensure there are no oils or dirt that could affect the application and longevity of the foundation.
- **Moisturize:** Apply a moisturizer suited to your skin type to hydrate and create a smoother surface. Allow it to absorb into the skin before applying makeup.
- **Prime:** Use a primer that addresses your specific skin concerns—such as mattifying, hydrating, or pore-minimizing. This helps create a seamless base and can extend the wear of your foundation.

2. Choosing the Right Foundation:

- **Shade Match:** Ensure the foundation matches your skin tone by testing it on your jawline, not your hand or wrist. The right shade should blend invisibly into your skin.
- **Undertone:** Pay attention to undertones; black skin can have cool, warm, or neutral undertones. Ensure your foundation complements this to avoid looking ashy or overly red.

- **Formula:** Consider your skin type and the coverage you need. Liquid foundations are versatile and work for most skin types, cream foundations offer dense coverage and work well for dry skin, while powder foundations are great for oily skin types.

3. Application Tools:

- **Beauty Sponge:** Use a damp beauty sponge for a dewy, natural finish. Bounce the sponge gently on the skin to blend the foundation without wiping it away.
- **Brush:** For fuller coverage, use a flat kabuki brush. Apply the foundation in circular motions to buff it into the skin, which helps achieve an airbrushed finish.
- **Fingers:** For those who prefer a lighter coverage or have very dry skin, fingers can be an effective tool. The warmth of your hands helps melt the foundation into the skin for a more natural look.

4. Application Technique:

- **Start Small:** Begin with a small amount of foundation in the center of the face, where most people need more coverage. Use less product on areas like the forehead and jawline where less coverage is typically needed.
- **Build Coverage:** Gradually add more foundation only where needed. Building up in thin layers helps maintain a natural look while providing sufficient coverage.
- **Blending:** Ensure all edges are blended seamlessly into the neck and hairline to avoid visible lines. Pay special attention to the nose and eye areas, where makeup can sometimes accumulate.

5. Setting the Foundation:

- **Setting Powder:** For oily skin types or to extend the wear of your foundation, apply a translucent setting powder with a fluffy brush. This helps to set the foundation and control shine.
- **Hydration:** For dry skin, consider using a hydrating mist after setting with powder to reduce any cakiness and add a luminous finish.

By following these steps, you can ensure your foundation looks flawless and stays in place throughout the day. Whether you're preparing for a day at work or a night out, these techniques will help you achieve a perfect base that enhances your natural beauty and complements your overall makeup look.

Concealer is a vital tool in any makeup routine, particularly for addressing under-eye circles, blemishes, and areas of hyperpigmentation. For black women, choosing the right concealer shade and formula is essential to achieve a flawless finish without ashiness or unnatural tones. Here's a detailed guide on how to apply concealer effectively.

1. Choosing the Right Concealer:

- **Color and Shade:** Select a concealer that matches your foundation for blemish and spot coverage. For brightening, especially under the eyes, choose a concealer one to two shades lighter than your skin tone.
- **Formula:** The formula should complement your skin type and the purpose of the concealer. Liquid concealers are versatile and great for under eyes and general coverage. Stick or cream concealers offer thicker coverage for blemishes and intense discoloration.

2. Preparation:

- **Hydrate:** Especially under the eyes, ensure the area is well-moisturized to prevent the concealer from looking cakey or settling into fine lines.
- **Prime:** Applying an eye primer can help in smoother application and increase the longevity of under-eye concealer.

3. Application for Under Eyes:

- **Apply in Triangles:** Instead of dotting concealer under the eyes, apply it in an inverted triangle shape with the base under your eye and the point toward your cheek. This technique helps create a natural-looking brightness that lifts the entire face.
- **Blend:** Use a damp beauty sponge or a soft brush to blend the concealer thoroughly. Ensure the edges are seamlessly integrated with your foundation to avoid visible lines.

4. Spot Concealing:

- **Precise Application:** Use a small concealer brush or a clean fingertip for precise application on blemishes, dark spots, or scars. Dab the concealer onto the spot and blend the edges without over-spreading the product, to maintain coverage.

- **Layer If Needed:** If the discoloration is still visible, let the first layer dry, then apply a second layer of concealer. Two thin layers often cover better than one thick layer.

5. Setting the Concealer:

- **Use Loose Powder:** To set the concealer, especially under the eyes, use a fine, loose setting powder. Apply with a small fluffy brush or a mini sponge, pressing the powder into the concealer to lock it in place without shifting the product.
- **Avoid Excess Powder:** Be cautious with the amount of powder; too much can dry out the skin and highlight fine lines. Just a light dusting is sufficient for setting the concealer.

6. Final Touches:

- **Blending with Overall Makeup:** Once the concealer is applied and set, go over the edges with a bit of your foundation on a sponge to ensure everything blends into a flawless complexion.
- **Reflective Light:** For additional brightness, especially in photography or special events, a light-reflective pen can be dabbed over the concealer under the eyes to enhance the illuminating effect.

Mastering the application of concealer not only improves the overall appearance of your makeup but also ensures that your complexion looks even and radiant throughout the day. By carefully selecting the right products and employing these techniques, you can effectively conceal imperfections and highlight your best features.

Tips for Long-Lasting Coverage

Ensuring that your foundation and concealer stay in place all day, particularly for black women who may experience issues with oiliness or makeup fading, requires specific techniques and products. Here's how to achieve long-lasting makeup coverage that remains fresh and flawless from morning until night.

1. Proper Skin Preparation:

- **Prime Well:** Always start with a primer tailored to your skin's needs. For oily skin, use a mattifying primer to control oil. For dry skin, a hydrating primer can prevent makeup from clinging to dry patches.
- **Moisturize:** Evenly moisturized skin is crucial for makeup adherence. Use an oil-free moisturizer if you have oily skin to keep the surface balanced.

2. Choose the Right Formulas:

- **Foundation:** Select a foundation that is long-wearing and suitable for your skin type. Foundations labeled as 'long-lasting' or '24-hour wear' are formulated to resist sweat, oil, and movement.
- **Concealer:** Opt for high-coverage, long-lasting concealers, especially for concealing blemishes or areas of hyperpigmentation.

3. Layering Techniques:

- **Thin Layers:** Apply makeup in thin layers, building up coverage gradually. Thick layers of makeup are more prone to sliding off or cracking.
- **Setting Spray Between Layers:** Mist a setting spray between each layer of makeup (post-primer, post-foundation, and post-concealer) to lock in each layer before applying the next.

4. Powder to Set:

- **Translucent Powder:** Use a loose, translucent setting powder to set your foundation and concealer. Apply it with a large, fluffy brush to avoid disrupting the makeup underneath.
- **Press and Roll:** For areas that need more solid setting, like the under-eye area or the T-zone, use a powder puff to press and roll the powder into the skin. This technique helps to mattify and smooth the skin effectively.

5. Blotting Throughout the Day:

- **Blotting Papers:** Instead of adding more powder throughout the day, which can lead to cakiness, use blotting papers to absorb excess oil without disturbing your makeup.

6. Touch-Up Smartly:

- **Minimal Product:** If you need to touch up, use a minimal amount of product. Too much can make the makeup look heavy. Ideally, dab a little concealer or foundation only on the areas that need it, then blend seamlessly.
- **Use Cream Products for Touch-Ups:** Cream products are easier to blend into existing makeup than powders. If you're refreshing your blush or bronzer, consider a cream formula.

7. Final Setting Spray:

- **Seal the Deal:** After all your makeup is applied, use a good quality setting spray. Choose one that suits your skin type: mattifying sprays for oily skin or hydrating sprays for dry skin.
- **Spray Technique:** Hold the bottle about 6-8 inches from your face and spritz in an X and T pattern to ensure even coverage.

By implementing these tips, your makeup coverage will not only look more polished and smooth but also last much longer. This approach is particularly effective for events, long workdays, or any time you need your makeup to look its best for extended periods.

In conclusion, this chapter has equipped you with the essential skills to expertly apply foundation and concealer, specifically catering to the unique requirements of black skin. The techniques and products highlighted here are designed to help you create a flawless base, tackle common concerns like oiliness and hyperpigmentation, and ensure your makeup lasts beautifully throughout the day. By understanding the importance of preparation, correct product selection, and effective application, you can enhance your natural beauty and feel confident in your makeup. Remember, practice is key to mastering these techniques, so I encourage you to experiment with the tips provided and discover what works best for you. Here's to achieving a stunning, long-lasting makeup look that celebrates and complements your individuality.

Chapter 6: Eye Makeup for Every Occasion

Eye makeup can define your look, whether you're aiming for a subtle day-time appearance or a dramatic evening presence. This chapter covers essential eye makeup techniques for different occasions, providing guidance tailored to enhance the unique beauty of darker skin tones.

Everyday Eye Makeup

For a simple and polished everyday look, it's important to choose techniques and colors that enhance your natural beauty without being too time-consuming or dramatic. This section provides step-by-step guidance on creating a flattering everyday eye makeup routine, particularly suited for darker skin tones.

Techniques and Color Recommendations:

- **Neutral Palette:** Opt for eyeshadows in neutral shades such as browns, beiges, and soft golds that complement your skin tone. These colors are subtle yet can define and enhance your eye shape beautifully.
- **Base Color:** Start by applying a light, matte shade all over the eyelid to even out the skin tone and provide a base for blending other colors.
- **Crease Definition:** Use a medium shade in the crease of your eyelid to add depth. For darker skin, warm medium browns work well to provide a soft contour without harshness.
- **Outer Corner:** To subtly enhance the eye shape, apply a slightly darker shade at the outer corner of the eye. Blend it well into the crease and along the lash line for a natural, seamless transition.

Application:

- **Eyeshadow Primer:** Begin with an eyeshadow primer to ensure your makeup stays put throughout the day without creasing. This step is crucial for maintaining a clean and vibrant look from morning to evening.
- **Lid Application:** Apply the light base color across the lid using a flat eyeshadow brush. This will help brighten the eye area and serve as a canvas for additional colors.

- **Crease Work:** With a fluffy blending brush, sweep the medium shade into the crease, using windscreen wiper motions to blend it out for a natural look. This step adds dimension without overt drama.
- **Outer V Definition:** Using a smaller, precise brush, apply the darkest shade to the outer corner of the eye in a 'V' shape and blend it towards the middle of the lid. This enhances the eye shape subtly but effectively.

Finishing Touches:

- **Eyeliner:** For an everyday look, opt for a soft eyeliner pencil in brown or black. Draw a thin line close to the upper lash line to define the eyes gently. Avoid heavy winged liner for this natural look.
- **Mascara:** Curl your lashes if desired, then apply one to two coats of mascara. Choose a volumizing formula to make your lashes look fuller without clumping. Ensure the mascara covers from the base to the tips of the lashes to open up the eye.
- **Optional Brow Filler:** Neatly groomed eyebrows frame the face and complement your eye makeup. Use a brow pencil or powder to fill in sparse areas, following the natural arch of your brows for a polished look.

This everyday eye makeup routine is designed to be both straightforward and flattering, providing a natural but defined appearance that's perfect for daily activities, whether you're heading to work, running errands, or meeting friends. By keeping the colors neutral and the application simple, you maintain a fresh and effortless beauty that enhances your natural features effectively.

Smokey Eye Tutorial

A smokey eye is a classic makeup look that's perfect for evenings out, special events, or whenever you want to add a bit of drama to your appearance. This tutorial will guide you through creating a smokey eye that is suitable for darker skin tones, ensuring the makeup enhances rather than overwhelms your features.

Step-by-Step Guide:

1. **Prime the Eyelids:**
   - Begin by applying an eyeshadow primer over the entire eyelid to ensure the makeup lasts longer and stays crease-free throughout the event.

2. **Base Color:**
   - Apply a neutral, matte eyeshadow slightly lighter than your skin tone all over your eyelid. This will help the darker shades blend more smoothly.
3. **Dark Shadow Application:**
   - Choose a dark eyeshadow—deep browns, dark grays, or blacks are ideal for a smokey look. Apply the shadow starting at the lash line and blend upwards towards the crease. Don't go too far beyond the crease as the look should remain concentrated on the lid and lower crease area.
4. **Blending:**
   - Use a clean, fluffy blending brush to soften any harsh lines. The key to a perfect smokey eye is seamless blending, so take your time to blend the dark shadow with the base color at the edges.
5. **Add Depth and Dimension:**
   - Apply a slightly shimmery or satin-finish eyeshadow in a dark tone to the center of the lid to add dimension. This step is optional but can enhance the smokey effect and add complexity to the look.
6. **Lower Lash Line:**
   - Using a small, precise brush, apply the same dark eyeshadow along the lower lash line. Smudge it out to match the top lid, creating a balanced and cohesive smokey effect.
7. **Eyeliner:**
   - Line your upper and lower waterlines with a black kohl eyeliner to intensify the smokey effect. You can also apply a gel or liquid liner along the top lash line to define the eyes further.
8. **Highlight the Inner Corner and Brow Bone:**
   - Apply a light, shimmery eyeshadow or a highlighter to the inner corners of your eyes and just beneath the arch of your brows. This brightens the overall look and makes the eyes pop.
9. **Mascara:**
   - Finish with several coats of volumizing mascara on both the top and bottom lashes to enhance the smokey eye. False lashes can also be added for an even more dramatic effect.

Tips for Dark Skin Tones:

- **Color Selection:** Darker skin tones can handle richer, more pigmented colors. Don't be afraid to use bold dark shades or even pops of color like navy or dark green for a unique take on the traditional smokey eye.
- **Matte vs. Shimmer:** While matte shadows are great for the smokey effect, incorporating a bit of shimmer can add depth and interest, especially under evening lights.

This smokey eye tutorial provides you with a structured approach to creating a captivating eye makeup look that can be tailored to fit any occasion. With practice, these steps will help you achieve a flawless and dramatic smokey eye that complements your darker skin tone beautifully.

Choosing Eyeshadows for Dark Skin Tones

Selecting the right eyeshadow shades is crucial for enhancing the beauty of dark skin tones. The right colors can make your eyes stand out and complement your complexion perfectly. This guide provides tips on choosing eyeshadows that enhance and complement dark complexions, ensuring vibrant, flattering eye makeup looks.

Understanding Color Theory:

- **Rich, Deep Shades:** Darker skin tones can beautifully carry rich and deep shades. Colors like deep purples, bold blues, and rich greens enhance the natural depth of your complexion.
- **Warm Colors:** Warm colors such as oranges, reds, and golds naturally complement dark skin by enhancing its natural glow.
- **Metallics:** Bronze, gold, copper, and metallic blues are particularly striking on darker skin tones. These shades add light and dimension to the eyes, making them pop.

Tips on Selecting Shades:

1. **Test Against Your Skin:** Always test eyeshadows against your skin tone, preferably in natural light. This will give you a true sense of how the color will look when applied.
2. **Pigmentation is Key:** Opt for eyeshadows that are highly pigmented. High-quality pigmentation ensures that the color shows up vividly on darker skin without having to apply too many layers.
3. **Consider Undertones:** Pay attention to your skin's undertones. If you have warm undertones, warm shades like gold and copper will look great. For cooler undertones, try cooler shades like deep blues and purples.
4. **Matte and Shimmer:** Include both matte and shimmer finishes in your collection. Matte shades are great for creating depth in the crease and defining the eye, while shimmer can be used on the lid or inner corner to highlight and brighten the eyes.

Building Your Palette:

- **Versatile Palette:** Create or choose a palette that includes both neutral and vibrant shades. This allows you to mix and match colors for daily wear and special occasions.
- **Transitional Shades:** Ensure you have good transitional shades (typically mid-toned colors) that can help blend darker shades into your skin tone seamlessly.
- **Highlight Colors:** Include lighter shades such as soft golds or light bronzes which can be used to highlight the brow bone and the inner corner of the eyes.

Application Tips:

- **Prime Your Lids:** Using an eyeshadow primer can make a significant difference in how pigmented the shadows appear on your skin. It helps the color adhere better and last longer, particularly important for darker skin tones.
- **Layering:** Start with lighter shades as a base and gradually build up to darker shades for a blended, cohesive look. Blending is crucial, so invest in good quality brushes that can help you seamlessly blend the colors.
- **Experiment:** Don't be afraid to experiment with colors and finishes. Sometimes, unexpected colors like a bright teal or a muted orange can look stunning when applied correctly.

Choosing eyeshadows for dark skin tones is all about embracing rich, pigmented colors that reflect your personal style and enhance your natural beauty. By understanding which shades complement your skin tone best, you can create eye makeup looks that are both striking and flattering.

Eyeliner and Mascara Tips for Stunning Eyes

Eyeliner and mascara are essential tools in any makeup arsenal, especially for creating eye looks that draw attention and highlight your best features. For dark skin tones, using these products effectively can accentuate the eyes dramatically. This guide offers tips and techniques for applying eyeliner and mascara to achieve stunning results.

Eyeliner Tips:

1. **Choosing the Right Color:**
   - **Classic Black:** A staple in any makeup kit, black eyeliner suits everyone and provides stark definition and contrast, especially on darker skin tones.

- ○ **Rich Browns:** A softer option than black, dark brown can offer a more subtle, natural look that still defines the eyes beautifully.
  - ○ **Vibrant Colors:** Don't shy away from bold colors like navy, forest green, or even metallics. These can highlight your eye color and add a fun element to your makeup.
2. **Application Techniques:**
  - ○ **Tightlining:** Applying eyeliner to the upper waterline adds intensity to your lash line, making your eyelashes appear thicker.
  - ○ **Winged Liner:** A well-executed wing can elongate the shape of your eyes and add a dramatic flair. Use a gel or liquid liner with a fine-tip brush for precision.
  - ○ **Smudged Look:** For a softer or smokey effect, use a pencil liner and smudge it slightly with a brush or smudger tool. This is great for a more casual or sultry look.
3. **Consider Your Eye Shape:**
  - ○ Adapt your eyeliner style to suit your eye shape. For example, those with smaller eyes should use thinner lines to avoid making eyes appear smaller, while those with larger eyes have more room to experiment with thicker and bolder lines.

Mascara Tips:

1. **Choosing the Right Mascara:**
  - ○ **Volume vs. Length:** Decide whether you want to add more volume or length. Thicker brushes are typically better for volume, while comb-like brushes are excellent for defining and lengthening.
  - ○ **Waterproof Formulas:** Consider a waterproof formula to prevent smudging throughout the day, especially if you have oily eyelids or live in a humid climate.
2. **Application Techniques:**
  - ○ **Wiggle the Wand:** To coat every lash evenly, start at the base of your lashes and wiggle the wand back and forth as you move toward the tips. This technique also helps prevent clumps.
  - ○ **Multiple Coats:** Apply two to three coats of mascara, allowing each coat to dry slightly (but not completely) between applications. This builds up volume and length without clumping.
  - ○ **Bottom Lashes:** Don't forget the bottom lashes. Use a lighter hand or even a different, more defining mascara to avoid overpowering your look.
3. **Curling Your Lashes:**
  - ○ **Use an Eyelash Curler:** Curling your lashes before applying mascara can make a significant difference, especially if your lashes tend to be

straight or point downwards. This step opens up your eyes and makes them appear larger and more awake.

By mastering these eyeliner and mascara techniques, you can enhance the natural beauty of your eyes, making them a captivating feature of your overall look. Whether aiming for a bold, dramatic style or a more understated chic appearance, these tips will help you create eye makeup that stands out beautifully against darker skin tones.

Chapter 7: Eyebrows and Lashes

Well-defined eyebrows and lush lashes can frame your face beautifully and enhance your overall makeup look. This chapter focuses on techniques for shaping and filling eyebrows, caring for your natural lashes, and applying false lashes effectively, tailored to complement dark skin tones.

Shaping and Filling Eyebrows

Well-defined eyebrows are essential for framing the face and enhancing overall facial aesthetics. This section provides detailed guidance on how to shape and fill eyebrows, particularly focusing on techniques that complement dark skin tones and ensure natural, polished results.

Shaping Eyebrows

1. **Assess Natural Brow Shape:**
    - Start by examining your natural eyebrows to determine their inherent shape and fullness. Identify any sparse areas or asymmetry that you might want to correct.
2. **Finding the Ideal Shape:**
    - **Start Point:** Align a straight object, like a makeup brush, vertically at the side of your nostril. Where the brush meets your brow is where your eyebrow should ideally start.
    - **Arch Point:** Angle the brush from the outside of your nostril through the pupil of your eye. The point where the brush intersects your eyebrow is where the arch should peak.
    - **End Point:** Angle the brush from the outside of your nostril to the outer corner of your eye. Where the brush meets the brow is where it should end.
3. **Trimming and Tweezing:**
    - Brush your eyebrows upward with a spoolie, and trim any hairs that are significantly longer than others to maintain a neat, even line.
    - Use tweezers to pluck stray hairs outside of your desired brow shape. Focus on cleaning up the area under the arch and between the brows to enhance your eyes and brighten your face.

Filling Eyebrows

1. **Choosing the Right Tools and Products:**
   - **Pencil:** Ideal for precise filling and defining. Choose a shade that matches your natural brow color or is one shade lighter.
   - **Powder:** Works well for a softer, more natural look. It's great for filling sparse areas without creating harsh lines.
   - **Gel:** Provides hold and adds color, perfect for thickening brows and setting them in place.
2. **Filling Technique:**
   - **Outline:** Lightly outline the lower border of your eyebrows with a pencil to define the shape. Avoid creating a harsh line; use light, short strokes to mimic natural hair.
   - **Fill Sparse Areas:** Use the pencil or powder to fill in gaps. Start at the sparsest part, usually at the arch or the tail, and work toward the front using the same short, hair-like strokes.
   - **Add Dimension:** If using powder, apply with a small angled brush for precision. Layer the color until you achieve the desired fullness and definition.
3. **Blending and Setting:**
   - **Blend:** Use a clean spoolie brush to blend the color through your brows. This softens any harsh lines and distributes the product evenly for a natural look.
   - **Set:** Apply a clear or tinted brow gel to set your brows in place. This helps control unruly hairs and keeps your filling product from fading or smudging throughout the day.

Tips for a Natural Look:

- Start filling your brows where they are most sparse, usually toward the middle or the end, and then use whatever product is left on the brush or pencil to lightly fill in the front of the brows. This keeps the look natural and avoids a stamped-on appearance.
- Consider the overall balance of your face when shaping your brows. Well-proportioned brows can help to harmonize facial features, making them a crucial aspect of your makeup routine.

By following these steps, you can achieve beautifully shaped and filled eyebrows that enhance your facial features and contribute to a polished makeup look. Whether you're preparing for a day at the office or a night out, well-defined eyebrows are key to looking your best.

Lash Care and Enhancement

Healthy and well-maintained eyelashes can significantly enhance your overall eye makeup and contribute to a more youthful and alert appearance. This section provides detailed tips on caring for your natural lashes and enhancing them through proper maintenance and the application of products designed specifically for lash health and beauty.

Daily Lash Care

1. **Gentle Cleansing:**
   - Always remove eye makeup at the end of the day using a gentle makeup remover. This prevents buildup, which can lead to lash breakage and loss.
   - Opt for oil-based removers for waterproof products, as they can dissolve makeup without excessive rubbing.
2. **Conditioning:**
   - Just like the hair on your scalp, eyelashes benefit from conditioning. Use a lash serum or natural oils (like castor oil, vitamin E oil, or coconut oil) at night to nourish and strengthen lashes.
   - Apply the oil or serum with a clean mascara wand or a cotton swab lightly to the lash line.

Promoting Lash Growth

1. **Lash Serums:**
   - Invest in a quality eyelash growth serum if you want to enhance your lash length and volume. These serums contain peptides and natural extracts to support lash growth and health.
   - Apply as directed, typically once a day, to clean, dry lashes.
2. **Healthy Diet:**
   - Lashes, like other hair, benefit from a balanced diet rich in vitamins and proteins. Foods high in vitamins C, E, and B-complex can help lashes grow thicker and stronger.

Mascara Application Techniques

1. **Choosing the Right Mascara:**

o   Select a mascara that suits your needs—lengthening, volumizing, or curling. For sensitive eyes, look for hypoallergenic formulas.
   o   Consider using a primer for lashes, which can help to extend the wear of your mascara and make your lashes appear fuller and longer.
2. **Application Tips:**
   o   Curl your lashes with an eyelash curler before applying mascara to open up the eyes and make lashes appear longer.
   o   Start at the base of your lashes and wiggle the wand slightly as you pull it through to the tips to separate the lashes and coat them evenly.
   o   Apply two coats for maximum impact, allowing the first coat to dry slightly before applying the second.

False Lashes for Enhancement

1. **Using False Lashes:**
   o   False lashes can be used for special occasions or to enhance your everyday look. Choose lashes that fit the natural shape and length of your own lashes for a more natural look, or go bold with longer, fuller versions for more drama.
   o   Trim the lashes to fit your eye shape before applying adhesive.
2. **Application:**
   o   Apply a thin line of lash glue to the band of the false lashes. Wait about 30 seconds for the glue to become tacky.
   o   Place the lashes as close to your natural lash line as possible using tweezers or a lash applicator for precision.
   o   Press down gently but firmly to secure them in place.

By following these tips for lash care and enhancement, you can ensure that your natural lashes remain healthy and that any enhancements look natural and appealing. Proper lash care can transform your overall eye makeup, making your eyes the standout feature of your face.

False Lashes Application

Applying false lashes can dramatically enhance your eye makeup, giving you a glamorous look suitable for special occasions or when you just want to feel extra fabulous. Here's a step-by-step guide to applying false lashes correctly, ensuring they look natural and stay secure throughout the day or night.

Choosing the Right False Lashes:

1. **Select a Style:**
   - Consider the occasion and the overall look you desire. For a natural look, choose lashes that are slightly longer than your natural lashes with a subtle curl. For a more dramatic effect, opt for thicker, fuller lashes.
   - Pay attention to the band; a thinner and more flexible band is easier to work with and feels more comfortable on the lid.
2. **Measure and Trim:**
   - Before applying glue, measure the false lashes against your natural lash line. If the lashes are too long, trim them from the outer edge to fit your eye shape better.

Preparing for Application:

1. **Curl Your Natural Lashes:**
   - Curl your natural lashes to match the curve of the false lashes. This step helps integrate your natural lashes with the falsies for a seamless look.
2. **Apply Mascara:**
   - Apply a coat of mascara to your natural lashes. This provides a sturdier base for the false lashes to adhere to and helps blend the natural and false lashes together.

Applying the Lashes:

1. **Apply Glue:**
   - Place a thin line of lash glue along the band of the false lashes. Let it dry for about 30 seconds or until the glue becomes tacky. This makes the lashes easier to stick without sliding around.
2. **Placement:**
   - Using tweezers or a lash applicator, place the false lashes as close as possible to your natural lash line. Start from the center, then adjust the ends. Press gently along the band to secure them in place.
   - Look down into a mirror placed on a flat surface; this angle makes it easier to apply lashes without blocking your view.

Securing and Blending:

1. **Secure the Corners:**
   - Make sure the corners are well-adhered to the skin. Press down gently but firmly with the end of the tweezers or your fingertips.
2. **Blend Lashes:**
   - Once the glue is dry, gently press your natural lashes and false lashes together with your fingers or the back of a makeup brush to blend them.

- If there is a visible gap between your natural lashes and the falsies, fill it in with a liquid eyeliner. This step also helps to hide any glue that might be showing.

Final Touches:

1. **Additional Mascara:**
   - Optionally, apply a light coat of mascara to further merge the natural and false lashes. However, be gentle to avoid clumping.
2. **Eyeliner Application:**
   - Apply eyeliner to the base of the lash line if needed to ensure everything looks seamless and to enhance the eye makeup.

By following these steps, you can master the art of false lash application, creating an eye-catching look that enhances your natural beauty. Proper application not only ensures that your lashes look great but also feel comfortable and stay in place as long as you need them to.

Chapter 8: Contouring and Highlighting for Deep Skin Tones

Contouring and highlighting are transformative makeup techniques that define and enhance facial features by playing with light and shadow. This chapter is dedicated to mastering these techniques for deep skin tones, ensuring that you can achieve a sculpted and luminous look that complements your natural beauty.

Understanding Contouring and Highlighting

Contouring and highlighting are advanced makeup techniques that enhance the structure of the face by defining features and adding dimension. These techniques are particularly effective on deep skin tones, as they can highlight natural beauty and create a balanced, radiant appearance. This section explains the fundamentals of contouring and highlighting, specifically tailored for those with darker complexions.

What is Contouring?

- **Definition and Purpose:** Contouring involves using makeup that is slightly darker than the skin tone to create shadows, which visually reshape and define areas of the face. For deep skin tones, contouring can emphasize cheekbones, slim the face, and sculpt the jawline.
- **Areas to Contour:** Common areas for contouring include under the cheekbones, along the hairline, the sides of the nose, and along the jawline. The goal is to enhance the natural face structure by deepening shadows.

What is Highlighting?

- **Definition and Purpose:** Highlighting is the opposite of contouring; it involves using lighter shades to bring certain features forward. This technique helps to illuminate the face, giving the skin a vibrant and youthful glow.
- **Areas to Highlight:** Key areas to highlight are the high points of the face where light naturally hits, such as the tops of the cheekbones, the bridge of the nose, the center of the forehead, the brow bones, and the cupid's bow above the upper lip.

The Synergy of Both Techniques:

- **Balanced Makeup:** When contouring and highlighting are done together, they create a harmonious balance. Contouring recedes areas you want to de-emphasize, while highlighting brings other areas forward. This balance is crucial for achieving a naturally sculpted look without appearing overly made-up.
- **Texture and Finish:** It's important to consider the finish of the products. Matte products are generally preferred for contouring to mimic the natural shadows, while shimmer or satin finishes are ideal for highlighters to reflect light.

Tips for Deep Skin Tones:

- **Shade Selection for Contouring:** Choose a contour shade that is one to two shades darker than your natural skin tone, with a cool or neutral undertone to mimic natural shadows effectively.
- **Highlighter Tones:** Opt for highlighters with gold, bronze, or copper undertones. These shades complement deep skin tones beautifully, adding warmth and glow without looking ashy.
- **Blending is Key:** Both contouring and highlighting require excellent blending to ensure there are no harsh lines or patches. This step is crucial for a seamless and natural look.

By understanding these concepts and applying them appropriately, individuals with deep skin tones can enhance their natural features in a way that is both subtle and impactful. Contouring and highlighting not only bring out your best features but also add depth and dimension to your overall makeup look, perfect for both everyday enhancement and special occasions.

Techniques for Defining Features

Contouring and highlighting are key makeup techniques used to define and enhance facial features by creating illusions of shadow and light. For deep skin tones, mastering these techniques can significantly elevate your makeup look by sculpting the face and bringing forward your best attributes. Here's a detailed guide on how to effectively use contouring and highlighting to define features.

Contouring Techniques:

1. **Preparation:**
   - Start with a well-prepped face. Ensure your skin is clean, moisturized, and primed to help the contour blend smoothly.

2. **Product Selection:**
   - Choose a contour product (cream, powder, or stick) that is one to two shades darker than your skin tone with a matte finish. The matte texture is crucial for creating the illusion of natural shadows.
3. **Application Areas and Methods:**
   - **Cheekbones:** To define cheekbones, suck in your cheeks to find the natural hollows. Apply the contour shade in the hollows from the ears towards the corners of your mouth, stopping midway. Blend upwards to lift the face.
   - **Jawline:** Enhance your jawline by applying contour along the jaw, blending downwards. This creates a shadow that sharpens and defines the jawline.
   - **Forehead:** If you have a high forehead, apply contour along the hairline to reduce the forehead's height. Blend upwards into the hairline for a natural effect.
   - **Nose:** For a slimmer nose, apply contour on the sides of the nose, blending it out carefully. A precise, small brush is ideal for this area.
4. **Blending:**
   - Use a blending brush or a damp beauty sponge to diffuse the edges of the contour. Ensure there are no harsh lines, and the transition between your foundation and contour is seamless.

Highlighting Techniques:

1. **Product Selection:**
   - Select a highlighter that complements your skin tone—typically gold, bronze, or rose gold tones work well with deep complexions. Opt for products with a smooth shimmer rather than chunky glitter.
2. **Application Areas and Methods:**
   - **Cheekbones:** Apply highlighter on the high points of your cheekbones. Blend towards the temples to create a lifted appearance.
   - **Brow Bone:** Highlight under the arch of your eyebrows to define your brow shape and enhance the eyes.
   - **Nose:** Apply a thin line of highlighter down the center of the nose to emphasize the nose's bridge. Be cautious with the amount to avoid an overly shiny appearance.
   - **Cupid's Bow:** A touch of highlighter on the cupid's bow can make your lips appear fuller and more defined.
3. **Blending Highlighter:**

o Use a fan brush or a tapered brush for a light and airy application. Ensure the highlighter blends into your base makeup without creating obvious lines.

Final Touches:

- **Set Your Makeup:** Use a setting spray to lock in your contour and highlight. This not only helps the makeup last longer but also melds the products together for a more natural look.
- **Final Assessment:** Check your makeup in different lighting to ensure it looks natural and the contours and highlights are effectively enhancing your features.

By following these contouring and highlighting techniques tailored for deep skin tones, you can sculpt your features in a way that enhances your natural beauty. This methodical approach ensures that you can achieve a polished and refined look, suitable for both everyday wear and special occasions.

Choosing the Right Products

Selecting the appropriate contouring and highlighting products is crucial for achieving a flawless makeup application that enhances and complements deep skin tones. The right shades and formulas can define and illuminate your facial features beautifully. This section guides you on how to choose the best products for contouring and highlighting if you have a deep complexion.

Choosing Contour Products:

1. **Shade Selection:**
   o **Right Shade:** Pick a contour shade that is one to two shades darker than your natural skin tone. The color should have a cool or neutral undertone to mimic the natural shadow your features would cast.
   o **Avoid Ashy Tones:** For deeper skin tones, it's important to choose shades that don't turn ashy. Bronzers with too much gray or overly light contour colors can appear muddy or ashy on darker skin.
2. **Formula:**
   o **Creams and Sticks:** Cream-based contours are ideal for dry skin or those who want a dewy finish. They blend easily and can be built up for more dramatic contouring.

- **Powders:** Powder contours work well for oily skin types and for those seeking a matte finish. They are also easier to control for subtle shading.
  - **Liquid Contours:** Liquid contours offer precision and are excellent for creating sharp, defined lines, especially around the nose and cheekbones.

Choosing Highlighting Products:

1. **Shade Selection:**
   - **Complementary Shades:** Choose highlighters with golden, bronze, or rose gold undertones that complement dark skin tones. These shades add a warm glow without appearing chalky.
   - **Test for Undertones:** Highlighters should enhance your skin, not contrast starkly. Avoid highlighters with too much silver or pale pink, which can look unnatural on deeper complexions.
2. **Formula:**
   - **Powder Highlighters:** These are great for oily skin or for those who prefer a subtle shimmer. They're easy to apply and blend out for a soft glow.
   - **Cream and Liquid Highlighters:** Ideal for dry skin, these formulas offer a dewy finish and tend to be more pigmented, providing a more intense glow. They can also be mixed with foundation for an all-over luminosity.
3. **Application Tools:**
   - **Brushes:** For powder products, use a fluffy, angled brush for contouring and a fan brush or tapered highlighter brush for highlighting. These tools help apply the product evenly and blend it out smoothly.
   - **Sponges and Fingers:** Cream and liquid products can be applied with a makeup sponge or fingers. These methods allow for more controlled blending, especially on smaller areas like the bridge of the nose or the brow bone.

Tips for Testing Products:

- **Swatch Before Buying:** Always swatch products on your skin, preferably in natural light, to see how they interact with your skin tone.
- **Consult Reviews and Tutorials:** Look for reviews and makeup tutorials by individuals with similar skin tones. This can provide insight into how products perform on deep skin tones.

Choosing the right contour and highlight products is about enhancing your natural beauty by creating depth and dimension. By selecting shades that mimic natural shadows and highlight areas where light naturally hits, you can ensure a natural, flattering look that enhances your deep skin tone beautifully.

Chapter 9: Blush and Bronzer

Blush and bronzer are essential components of a makeup routine, especially for dark skin tones, as they add warmth, dimension, and a healthy glow to the complexion. This chapter will guide you through selecting the right shades and applying blush and bronzer for a natural, flattering look on darker skin.

Selecting Shades that Compliment Dark Skin

Choosing the right shades of makeup, particularly blush and bronzer, is crucial for enhancing the natural beauty of dark skin tones. The correct shades will blend seamlessly with the skin, adding warmth, dimension, and a radiant glow. This section provides guidance on selecting shades that compliment darker complexions effectively.

Blush for Dark Skin:

1. **Rich, Vibrant Colors:**
    - **Deep Reds and Berries:** These shades are highly pigmented and can give a natural flushed look that is visible and flattering on darker skin.
    - **Warm Browns and Tangerines:** Such colors mimic the natural warmth of darker skin and can enhance the complexion without overwhelming it.
2. **Experiment with Undertones:**
    - Consider blushes with different undertones to see what highlights your skin best. Shades with gold or bronze undertones can also double as a light bronzer, giving a glowy effect.
3. **Texture and Finish:**
    - Both matte and shimmer finishes can work well, but it's important to consider the overall makeup look. Matte blushes provide a more natural finish, while shimmer can add a radiant glow, perfect for evening looks.

Bronzer for Dark Skin:

1. **Golden and Copper Tones:**
    - Look for bronzers that are warm with a golden or copper base. These tones add a natural sun-kissed warmth to the skin.
    - Avoid anything too light or with a grey undertone, as it can appear muddy or ashy.
2. **Depth and Dimension:**

- The bronzer should be just a shade or two darker than your natural skin tone. It should add definition and a subtle contour to the face, not an overt color change.
3. **Formula Preferences:**
   - Powder bronzers are great for oily skin and achieving a matte finish. Cream or liquid bronzers blend well on dry or combination skin and offer a dewy look.

Testing and Matching:

- **Swatch Before Buying:** Always swatch cosmetics on your skin, ideally along the jawline or on the back of your hand, to see how the product melds with your skin under natural light.
- **Consultations:** If possible, consult with a makeup expert who has experience with dark skin tones. They can offer personalized advice and product recommendations.

Additional Tips:

- **Blending is Key:** No matter the color or product, proper blending is essential. Well-blended makeup looks natural and highlights your features more effectively.
- **Layering Products:** Don't be afraid to layer different products. For example, layering a matte bronzer under a shimmer blush can create a beautifully nuanced effect.

Selecting the right shades for blush and bronzer is more than just picking the darkest or the brightest options available; it's about finding hues that naturally enhance and complement your skin tone. By following these guidelines, individuals with dark skin can choose products that will highlight their natural beauty and contribute to a flawless makeup application.

Application Tips for a Natural Look

Achieving a natural makeup look, especially when using products like blush and bronzer on dark skin tones, involves using the right techniques to apply these products subtly and effectively. This guide provides essential tips on how to apply blush and bronzer to enhance your natural beauty without looking overdone.

Blush Application Tips:

1. **Select the Right Brush:**
   - Use a fluffy, medium-sized blush brush for the application. This type of brush helps distribute the product evenly, avoiding harsh lines.
2. **Technique for a Natural Flush:**
   - Smile to find the apples of your cheeks. Lightly apply blush to the apples and blend upwards towards the temples. This placement mimics a natural flush.
   - Start with a light hand, building up color gradually. It's easier to add more product than to take it away.
3. **Blending:**
   - After applying blush, use a clean brush or a beauty sponge to softly blend the edges into your foundation. This step ensures there are no obvious lines and the blush looks like it's coming from beneath the skin.
4. **Choosing Colors:**
   - Opt for colors that mimic a natural flush. On dark skin, rich reds, deep oranges, and berry shades can look incredibly natural and vibrant.

Bronzer Application Tips:

1. **Select the Right Brush:**
   - Use a large, fluffy brush for bronzer application. A bigger brush helps apply the product lightly and evenly, which is key for a natural look.
2. **Technique for Subtle Definition:**
   - Apply bronzer to areas where the sun naturally hits the face: the perimeter of the forehead, just below the cheekbones, and along the jawline.
   - Use the "3" shape technique: start from the forehead, bring the brush in a curve to below the cheekbones, and then down another curve to below the jawline. This method ensures a harmonious application that enhances your facial structure.
3. **Blending:**
   - Blend thoroughly to avoid any harsh lines or patches. The goal is for the bronzer to provide warmth and slight contouring without looking like makeup.
4. **Layering and Balancing:**
   - Balance the warmth of the bronzer with a neutral setting powder if necessary to maintain a natural appearance. Lightly dust setting powder in the center of the face to keep the focus on the contoured areas.

Combining Both Products:

- **Harmony Between Blush and Bronzer:**
    - Ensure that the blush and bronzer blend into each other without distinct boundaries. Use a clean fluffy brush to meld the edges where the blush and bronzer meet.
    - Consider the overall tone and effect; the blush should add a pop of color, while the bronzer adds warmth and definition.

By following these application tips, you can create a natural-looking makeup effect that enhances your skin tone and features without overwhelming them. The key to a natural look is subtlety and blending, ensuring that each product complements rather than competes with the other. This approach is particularly effective for darker skin tones, where well-chosen blush and bronzer can dramatically enhance the complexion's natural radiance.

Chapter 10: Lips

Achieving beautiful, well-defined lips can transform your entire makeup look. This chapter is dedicated to lip care, selecting the right colors, and applying lipstick techniques specifically tailored for fuller, more striking lips. These tips are particularly beneficial for individuals looking to enhance and highlight their lips as a key feature of their makeup routine.

Lip Care Basics

Proper lip care is essential for maintaining healthy, soft, and smooth lips, especially important as a foundation for beautiful makeup application. Here are fundamental steps and tips to ensure your lips are well cared for, enhancing their natural beauty and preparing them for any lip color application.

Regular Exfoliation:

1. **Why It's Important:**
   - Regular exfoliation helps remove dead skin cells from the lips, preventing dryness and flakiness. This is crucial for keeping lips smooth and ready for an even application of lip products.
2. **How to Exfoliate:**
   - Use a gentle lip scrub once or twice a week. You can easily make a homemade scrub with sugar mixed with honey or olive oil for a natural, effective treatment.
   - Alternatively, you can use a soft toothbrush with a bit of lip balm to gently brush over the lips. This not only exfoliates but also stimulates blood flow, making lips appear fuller and more vibrant.

Hydration:

1. **Daily Lip Moisturizing:**
   - Apply a hydrating lip balm regularly throughout the day. Choose balms that contain emollients and humectants like shea butter, beeswax, vitamin E, and hyaluronic acid. These ingredients help lock in moisture and protect the lips from environmental factors.
   - Before bed, apply a thicker layer of a nourishing lip treatment or balm to repair your lips overnight.
2. **Drinking Water:**

- Keeping hydrated is essential for maintaining overall health, including the health of your lips. Drink plenty of water throughout the day to help keep your lips (and skin) hydrated from the inside out.

Protection:

1. **Sun Protection:**
   - Lips are vulnerable to sun damage, which can lead to dryness and premature aging. Use lip products that contain SPF to protect against UVA and UVB rays, especially if you are going to be outdoors.
   - Reapply sunscreen-containing products every two hours when exposed to sunlight.

Avoid Harmful Habits:

1. **Don't Lick Your Lips:**
   - Avoid licking your lips. While it might feel like a quick fix for dryness, saliva evaporates quickly, taking more moisture from your lips and leaving them drier than before.
   - Saliva also contains enzymes that can irritate the delicate skin around the lips.
2. **Healthy Diet:**
   - A diet rich in vitamins and minerals supports healthy skin and lips. Ensure you consume foods high in vitamins A, C, E, and omega-3 fatty acids, which contribute to strong, resilient skin.

By incorporating these lip care basics into your daily routine, you can ensure that your lips remain healthy, hydrated, and smooth. Proper lip care not only improves the appearance of your lips but also enhances the performance and finish of any lip color you apply, contributing to a more polished and beautiful makeup look.

Choosing Lip Colors

Selecting the right lip color is crucial for complementing your overall makeup look and enhancing your natural beauty, especially for individuals with deep skin tones. Here's a guide on how to choose lip colors that not only suit your skin tone but also fit various occasions and personal styles.

Understanding Skin Undertones:

1. **Identify Your Undertone:**
   - Determine whether your skin has warm, cool, or neutral undertones. This can impact which shades will look best on you. Warm undertones look great with warm colors like red, orange, and coral. Cool undertones are complemented by blue-based colors like pink, berry, and mauve. Neutral undertones can usually pull off a wide range of colors.
2. **Complementing Deep Skin Tones:**
   - Rich, deep colors generally look stunning on darker skin tones. Experiment with bold shades such as deep reds, purples, and vibrant berries.
   - Don't shy away from nudes; choose nudes with hints of brown or pink to enhance your natural lip color without washing you out.

Selecting Shades for Different Occasions:

1. **Everyday Wear:**
   - Opt for lighter or more neutral shades for daytime or casual settings. Soft pinks, peaches, and light browns can be perfect for a natural, understated look.
2. **Work Environment:**
   - Choose more conservative shades that add a touch of color without being too bold. Mauves, rosy pinks, and subtle reds can be professional yet stylish.
3. **Evening and Special Events:**
   - Go bold with darker or brighter colors for evenings or special occasions. Deep reds, vibrant pinks, or even metallic finishes can make a strong statement and elevate your evening wear.

Experimenting with Textures and Finishes:

1. **Matte:**
   - Matte lipsticks offer intense color payoff and long-lasting wear. They work well for both formal and high-impact looks but can be drying, so make sure your lips are well-moisturized before application.
2. **Cream and Satin:**
   - These finishes provide a slight sheen, offering a balance between matte and gloss. They are generally more hydrating and suitable for everyday wear.
3. **Gloss:**

- Lip glosses are perfect for adding shine and can be used alone for a subtle look or over a lipstick to add dimension. They make lips appear fuller and more plump.

Tips for Choosing and Using Lip Color:

- **Test Before Buying:** Whenever possible, test the lipstick on your lips rather than just swatching it on your hand. This will give you a better idea of how it looks with your natural lip color and skin tone.
- **Consider Your Wardrobe:** Think about the colors you typically wear. Choosing lipstick shades that coordinate with your wardrobe can help create a cohesive and polished look.
- **Personal Preference:** Ultimately, the best lip color is one that makes you feel confident and beautiful. Don't be afraid to try new shades and textures that might seem unconventional. Makeup is a form of self-expression!

By understanding how to select the right lip colors and finishes for your skin tone and occasions, you can enhance your makeup routine and express your personal style confidently.

Application Techniques for Full, Beautiful Lips

Creating the illusion of fuller, more defined lips is an art that can be mastered with the right techniques and tools. This guide provides detailed steps for applying lip products in a way that enhances the natural beauty of your lips, making them appear plumper and more striking, especially on darker skin tones.

Preparing Your Lips:

1. **Exfoliation and Hydration:**
   - Start by exfoliating your lips with a gentle lip scrub to remove any flaky skin. This ensures a smooth canvas for lipstick application.
   - Apply a hydrating lip balm and let it absorb for a few minutes. Blot any excess with a tissue to prevent the lipstick from slipping.

Lining Your Lips:

1. **Choose the Right Lip Liner:**

- Select a lip liner that closely matches your lipstick shade. Liner helps define the lips and creates a boundary that prevents lipstick from bleeding.

2. **Outline and Fill:**
   - Carefully outline your natural lip line, starting from the cupid's bow and moving outward. You can slightly overline at the cupid's bow and beneath the center of the lower lip to create the illusion of fullness, but keep the lines realistic to avoid an overdone look.
   - Fill in the entire lip with the liner to help the lipstick last longer and fade more evenly.

Applying Lipstick:

1. **Application Technique:**
   - Apply your lipstick directly from the tube or use a lip brush for more precision, especially with bold or dark shades.
   - Start at the center of your lips and work outwards, filling in all areas. A lip brush can help you get into the corners and fine-tune the edges.
2. **Blot and Reapply:**
   - Blot your lips with a piece of tissue to remove excess oil and then apply a second layer. This helps set the first layer and adds longevity and intensity to the color.
3. **Highlight for Fullness:**
   - Add a tiny dab of highlighter or a lighter lipstick shade to the center of your bottom lip and cupid's bow. This trick catches the light, making your lips look fuller.

Final Touches:

1. **Clean the Edges:**
   - Use a small brush dipped in concealer to clean up the edges around your lips. This not only sharpens the lines but also helps highlight the lips, making them stand out more.
2. **Set with Powder:**
   - If you prefer a matte finish, lightly dust translucent powder over your lips through a tissue. This sets the lipstick without altering the color.
3. **Gloss for Added Volume:**
   - For added fullness, apply a clear or matching lip gloss over your lipstick, focusing on the center of the lips. Gloss reflects light, adding a voluminous effect.

By following these application techniques, you can enhance the natural shape and size of your lips, creating a fuller, more defined look that complements your overall makeup. Whether you're aiming for a subtle enhancement or a dramatic evening look, these steps will help you achieve beautiful, impactful lips.

Chapter 11: Setting Your Makeup

Setting your makeup properly is essential to ensure it stays in place and looks fresh all day or night. This chapter provides a comprehensive guide on how to choose and use setting powders and sprays effectively, along with tips to maximize the longevity of your makeup, particularly beneficial for those with deeper skin tones.

Choosing Setting Powders and Sprays

Choosing Setting Powders and Sprays

Selecting the right setting powders and sprays is crucial for achieving a flawless makeup finish that lasts all day or night. These products help to lock in your makeup, control shine, and ensure your look remains fresh. Here's how to choose the best setting powders and sprays, especially for those with deeper skin tones.

Choosing Setting Powders

1. **Consider Your Skin Tone:**
   - **For Dark Skin Tones:** Choose a setting powder that matches your skin tone or opt for a translucent formula. Avoid powders that are too light as they can leave a white cast or appear ashy.
   - **Colored vs. Translucent:** Colored powders can add a little extra coverage and even out skin tone, while translucent powders are designed to set makeup without adding color.
2. **Texture and Finish:**
   - **Finely Milled Powders:** Look for ultra-fine powders that blend seamlessly into the skin. These are less likely to clump or settle into fine lines and pores.
   - **Matte vs. Dewy:** Choose a matte finish powder if you have oily skin or prefer a shine-free finish. For drier skin or those who want a more natural, radiant finish, look for powders that offer a luminous effect without being glittery.

Choosing Setting Sprays

1. **Based on Skin Type:**
   - **Mattifying Sprays:** Ideal for oily skin, these sprays help control excess oil and reduce shine throughout the day.

- ○ **Hydrating Sprays:** Perfect for dry or normal skin, hydrating sprays can refresh makeup and add a dewy glow. They often contain ingredients like glycerin or hyaluronic acid.
2. **Consider the Ingredients:**
   - ○ **Alcohol-Free Options:** If you have sensitive or dry skin, avoid setting sprays that contain high amounts of alcohol, which can be drying.
   - ○ **Skin-Beneficial Ingredients:** Look for sprays enriched with vitamins, minerals, and antioxidants to provide additional skincare benefits.
3. **Spray Mechanism:**
   - ○ **Fine Mist:** Ensure the setting spray bottle delivers a fine, even mist. This prevents droplets that can cause makeup to run or look patchy. Test the spray before buying if possible.

Application Tips:

- **How to Apply Setting Powder:**
  - ○ Use a large, fluffy brush for a light, even application or a makeup sponge to press the powder into areas that need more oil control.
  - ○ Focus on areas prone to oiliness or where makeup tends to break down, such as the T-zone, under the eyes, and around the nose.
- **How to Apply Setting Spray:**
  - ○ Shake the bottle well, hold it several inches away from your face, and spray in an "X" and "T" pattern to cover all areas evenly.
  - ○ Allow the spray to dry naturally for the best results.

By choosing the right setting powders and sprays for your skin type and tone, and applying them correctly, you can significantly enhance the longevity and quality of your makeup. This ensures a polished look that remains stable throughout the day or evening, highlighting your features beautifully without frequent touch-ups.

Tips for Long-Lasting Wear

Ensuring your makeup remains flawless throughout the day involves more than just the initial application. Here are essential tips for achieving long-lasting wear, which will help your makeup stay fresh, vibrant, and intact for hours, regardless of your activities or the environment.

Preparation is Crucial:

1. **Skin Care Foundation:**
   - **Start with Clean Skin:** Always begin with a clean face. Excess oil, dirt, or residual makeup can affect how new products adhere and last on your skin.
   - **Moisturize Appropriately:** Use a moisturizer suitable for your skin type. This helps to create a smooth canvas and prevents makeup from clinging to dry patches or becoming oily.
2. **Use a Primer:**
   - **Face Primer:** Apply a primer that addresses your skin concerns (e.g., pore-minimizing, hydrating, mattifying). Primer can significantly extend the wear of your makeup by providing a barrier between oil production and your foundation.
   - **Eye Primer:** Don't forget the eyelids. Using an eye primer prevents eyeshadow from creasing and helps pigments appear more vibrant.

Application Techniques:

1. **Layer Thinly:**
   - Build coverage with thin layers of foundation or concealer. Thick layers are more prone to sliding off or creasing. Allow each layer to set before applying the next.
2. **Use Long-Wear Formulas:**
   - Invest in high-quality, long-wear makeup products. These are specifically formulated to resist sweat, oil, and friction.
3. **Setting Properly:**
   - **Powder:** After applying liquid or cream foundations and concealers, set your makeup with a fine, loose setting powder. This absorbs excess oil and locks the base in place.
   - **Spray:** Finish with a setting spray. Choose a formula that suits your skin type and makeup finish preference. This step seals the makeup and can also refresh the skin.

Throughout the Day:

1. **Blotting Papers:**
   - Use blotting papers to manage oil and shine throughout the day. Blotting helps to absorb excess oil without disrupting your makeup.
2. **Touch-Ups:**
   - Carry a compact powder or a small concealer for quick touch-ups. These are particularly useful for refreshing makeup under the eyes or around the nose.

3. **Hydration:**
   - Keep your skin hydrated from the inside by drinking plenty of water. This not only benefits your overall health but also helps maintain the skin's moisture balance, improving makeup longevity.

External Factors:

1. **Environmental Considerations:**
   - Be mindful of environmental factors such as heat, humidity, and wind. Use appropriate products that can withstand these conditions, such as waterproof mascaras or extra-hold setting sprays.
2. **Lifestyle:**
   - Consider your daily activities. If you have a physically demanding job or tend to touch your face frequently, you may need to invest in stronger, more durable makeup products or adjust your application techniques to ensure longer wear.

By implementing these tips, you can significantly improve the longevity of your makeup, ensuring it stays put and looks great from morning till night. Preparation, smart product choices, and occasional touch-ups will help maintain your look, no matter what your day entails.

Chapter 12: Special Occasion Makeup

Special occasions demand a more elevated makeup approach to ensure you look your best, whether for a wedding, a gala evening, or a professional photoshoot. This chapter will guide you through creating stunning looks tailored to each event, focusing on techniques that enhance and celebrate your features.

Wedding Makeup

Wedding makeup is an integral part of a bride's big day, designed to enhance her natural beauty and ensure she looks flawless from the ceremony to the last dance. For Black women, choosing the right makeup involves not only embracing their style and personality but also highlighting their rich skin tones and textures. Here's a comprehensive guide to achieving a beautiful, long-lasting wedding makeup look that will stand out both in person and in photos.

Foundation and Base

Start with a high-quality, long-wearing foundation that matches the skin tone perfectly and offers buildable coverage. It should be resistant to smudging and fading, and ideally free of SPF to avoid flashback in photography. Use a primer that complements the bride's skin type—be it hydrating, mattifying, or smoothing—to ensure a smooth application and extend the durability of the foundation. Apply a lightweight, crease-resistant concealer under the eyes and on any blemishes or redness, blending thoroughly for a seamless finish. Set the makeup with a fine, translucent powder, focusing on areas prone to oiliness like the T-zone to minimize shine and keep the base in place.

Eyes

Opt for classic, soft eyeshadow shades such as neutral browns, soft pinks, or gentle golds, which work well with most wedding themes and beautifully enhance the bride's eye color. Add a slight shimmer on the lids for a bright, open-eyed look, avoiding overly glittery formulas. Use a waterproof gel or liquid eyeliner to create a defined look, possibly adding a subtle wing to lift and elongate the eyes. Apply waterproof mascara to ensure the look holds through emotional moments, and consider natural-looking false lashes to enhance volume and length without being overly dramatic.

Cheeks and Contour

Choose a blush that complements the natural flush of the cheeks. Cream blushes are ideal for blending into a dewy, natural glow. Apply the blush on the apples of the cheeks and blend upwards towards the temples to lift the face. For contouring, use a matte bronzer or contour powder to subtly define the cheekbones and jawline, enhancing facial features softly and avoiding harsh lines.

Lips

Select a lip color that complements the overall makeup—popular choices include soft pinks, corals, or nudes. Start by applying a lip liner in a matching shade to define the lips and prevent color bleeding. Opt for a long-wearing lipstick formula, preferably in a matte finish for its durability. Ensure the lips are well-moisturized before applying lipstick to maintain comfort and prevent cracking.

Final Touches

Finish the makeup application with a setting spray that suits the desired finish, whether matte or dewy, to help lock the makeup in place. Hold the spray at arm's length and mist lightly, allowing it to dry naturally. Prepare a small touch-up kit for the bride that includes blotting papers, lipstick, and a mini powder compact for quick fixes throughout the day.

By following these steps, you can ensure the bride's makeup is not only beautiful but also functional, maintaining its elegance and style throughout a day filled with significant moments. This approach highlights current trends favoring vibrant colors and matte finishes, while ensuring the makeup enhances rather than overshadows the bride's natural beauty, offering a look that is radiant and elegantly defined.

Evening and Gala Makeup

Evening and gala events often call for a more dramatic and polished makeup look that stands out in a crowd and complements formal attire. This guide will walk you through creating a sophisticated and elegant evening makeup look, perfect for galas, formal dinners, or any nighttime event where you want to make a statement.

Foundation and Base:

1. **Flawless Foundation:**

- Opt for a full-coverage foundation that provides a smooth and even canvas. Evening lighting and photography demand a flawless finish that hides imperfections and enhances your natural complexion.
    - Use a mattifying primer if you have oily skin, or a hydrating primer for dry skin, to ensure the foundation adheres well and stays put throughout the event.
2. **Concealer:**
    - Apply a high-coverage concealer to address under-eye circles and any blemishes or redness. Make sure to blend seamlessly with the foundation for a uniform look.
3. **Setting Powder:**
    - Use a translucent setting powder to set your foundation, paying extra attention to the T-zone and under-eye area to prevent creasing and shine.

Eyes:

1. **Dramatic Eyeshadow:**
    - Choose richer, deeper shades like dark browns, smoky grays, or jewel tones such as emerald or sapphire. These colors add depth and drama appropriate for evening wear.
    - Consider incorporating a shimmer or metallic finish on the lids to catch the light and add dimension.
2. **Eyeliner and Mascara:**
    - Use a black waterproof eyeliner for a sharp and defined eye look. A winged eyeliner can elevate the sophistication of your makeup.
    - Apply multiple coats of volumizing or lengthening mascara, or opt for dramatic false lashes to accentuate and open up the eyes.

Cheeks:

1. **Contour and Highlight:**
    - Sculpt your face with a contour powder or cream slightly darker than your skin tone. Focus on the hollows of your cheeks, sides of the nose, and jawline.
    - Use a luminous highlighter on the high points of your face such as cheekbones, brow bones, and down the center of the nose to create a radiant glow.
2. **Blush:**

- o Apply a blush with a hint of shimmer to the apples of your cheeks and blend upwards towards the temples. Choose a color that complements the overall tone of your makeup and adds warmth to your complexion.

Lips:

1. **Bold Lip Color:**
   - o Evening events are the perfect occasion to wear bold lip colors. Choose deep reds, vibrant berries, or rich plums to make a statement.
   - o Line your lips with a matching lip liner before applying your lipstick to ensure precision and to prevent the color from bleeding. Fill in the lips with the liner for added longevity.
2. **Matte or Glossy Finish:**
   - o Decide between a matte finish for longevity and a classic look, or a glossy finish for a plump, attention-grabbing effect.

Final Touches:

1. **Setting Spray:**
   - o Finish your makeup with a setting spray that suits your skin type and the desired finish (matte or dewy). This will help lock everything in place and ensure your makeup lasts all night.
2. **Touch-Up Kit:**
   - o Consider bringing a small touch-up kit with your lipstick, a small mirror, and blotting papers to maintain your look throughout the event.

By following these steps, you can create a stunning evening makeup look that is both glamorous and enduring, ensuring you look your best for any gala or evening event.

Makeup for Photoshoots

Makeup for photoshoots requires precise application and strategic choices to ensure it looks perfect under various lighting conditions and through the lens of a camera. This guide covers essential tips for creating a camera-ready look that will photograph beautifully and enhance the subject's features effectively.

Foundation and Base:

1. **High Definition Foundation:**
   - Use a high-definition or photo-friendly foundation that offers seamless coverage without a flashback effect. These foundations are designed to look natural and flawless on camera.
   - Avoid foundations with SPF as they can create a white cast in photos due to their light-reflective properties.
2. **Concealer:**
   - Apply a full-coverage concealer to hide any imperfections, dark circles, or blemishes. Blending is key to ensure there are no visible lines or color discrepancies under studio lighting.
3. **Setting Powder:**
   - Opt for a finely milled, translucent setting powder to set the makeup. This helps to minimize shine and maintain the foundation's finish throughout the shoot.

Eyes:

1. **Eye Makeup Considerations:**
   - Eye makeup should be slightly more defined for photoshoots as features tend to look less pronounced in photos. Use deeper shades to define the eye crease and lash lines.
   - Matte shadows are preferable for most professional photos as they reduce glare. Add just a touch of shimmer on the center of the lids to make the eyes pop without causing excessive shine.
2. **Eyeliner and Mascara:**
   - Waterproof and smudge-proof eyeliner is essential, especially for long shoots or those involving action scenes. A gel liner usually offers a precise and lasting application.
   - Multiple coats of waterproof mascara will define the lashes. Consider false lashes to dramatically enhance the eyes, especially for close-up shots.

Cheeks:

1. **Contour and Highlight:**
   - Contouring should be strategic and not too heavy. Use a shade that naturally shadows the face to sculpt the cheekbones, jawline, and temples.
   - Highlight should be subtle and placed on the high points of the face where light naturally hits. Avoid overly glittery highlighters as they can create undesirable reflections.

2. **Blush:**
   - Use a blush that enhances the skin tone and complements the overall makeup theme. Blend well to ensure the color looks natural and consistent under different lighting.

Lips:

1. **Lip Color:**
   - Choose lip colors that stand out and complement the overall makeup palette. Matte lipsticks are often preferred for their long-lasting properties and minimal transfer.
   - Outline the lips with a matching lip liner before applying lipstick to define the shape and prevent bleeding.

Final Preparations:

1. **Matte Finish:**
   - Given that high-shine can distract in photographs, aim for a matte finish across the skin. Use blotting sheets to remove excess oil without disturbing the makeup.
2. **Final Touch-Ups:**
   - Prior to shooting, do a final check with a hand mirror in both natural and artificial lighting to ensure makeup looks consistent and flawless from every angle.
3. **Setting Spray:**
   - A light mist of setting spray can lock in the makeup and reduce the need for frequent touch-ups, which is especially important during longer photoshoots.

By adhering to these guidelines, makeup artists can ensure that the makeup not only looks spectacular in person but also translates beautifully and effectively on camera, perfect for any photoshoot scenario.

Chapter 13: Troubleshooting Common Makeup Issues

Even the most carefully applied makeup can encounter issues throughout the day or under different conditions. This chapter provides solutions to common makeup problems, helping you manage oiliness, correct makeup mishaps, and adjust your look for various lighting scenarios.

Managing Oiliness Throughout the Day

Controlling oiliness throughout the day is a common challenge, especially for those with naturally oily skin types. Effective management can ensure your makeup stays fresh and matte without frequent touch-ups. Here are strategies to help keep your skin looking its best from morning till evening.

Start with the Right Base:

1. **Use a Mattifying Primer:**
   - Begin your makeup routine with a mattifying primer. This product helps to control oil production and creates a smooth, matte surface that enhances the longevity of your foundation.
2. **Choose Oil-Free Foundations:**
   - Opt for oil-free and non-comedogenic foundation formulas. These are specifically designed to prevent pore clogging and reduce the shine that can develop throughout the day.

Set with Powder:

1. **Translucent Setting Powder:**
   - After applying foundation and concealer, use a translucent setting powder to set your makeup. Focus on areas prone to oiliness, such as the T-zone (forehead, nose, and chin).
   - Apply the powder with a fluffy brush for a light coverage or use a puff to press the powder into the skin for a more durable matte finish.
2. **Consider Powder Formulas:**
   - If your skin is extremely oily, consider using mineral or powder foundations instead of liquid types. These can help absorb oil naturally throughout the day.

Blotting Techniques:

1. **Use Blotting Papers:**
   - Carry blotting papers with you. These are great for quick touch-ups and to remove excess oil without disturbing your makeup. Gently press a blotting paper against oily areas instead of rubbing.
2. **Touch Up Strategically:**
   - After blotting, if you notice any makeup has worn off, use a small amount of pressed powder to touch up. Avoid adding too much product, which can lead to cakiness.

Additional Tips:

1. **Avoid Over-Moisturizing:**
   - If you have oily skin, use a lightweight or gel-based moisturizer. Over-moisturizing can trigger more oil production.
2. **Setting Sprays:**
   - Finish your makeup with an oil-control setting spray. These sprays are designed to seal your makeup and can significantly extend wear time by reducing oiliness.
3. **Regular Skincare Routine:**
   - Maintain a regular skincare routine that addresses oil control. Products containing salicylic acid or niacinamide can be effective at managing oil production and keeping pores clear.

By implementing these techniques, you can help control oil production throughout the day, ensuring your makeup remains fresh, matte, and flawless for longer periods. Regularly monitoring and adjusting your skincare and makeup routine according to your skin's needs will also contribute significantly to managing oiliness effectively.

Quick Fixes for Makeup Mishaps

Even with the best application techniques, makeup mishaps can happen. Knowing how to quickly and efficiently correct these errors can save your look and your day. Here are some essential tips for addressing common makeup mistakes, ensuring your makeup remains flawless.

Fixing Smudged Eyeliner or Mascara:

1. **Cotton Swab and Makeup Remover:**
    - Dip a cotton swab in makeup remover and gently clean up any smudges from eyeliner or mascara. This precise tool allows you to target just the mistake without disturbing the rest of your makeup.
    - If you remove a bit of foundation or concealer in the process, dab a tiny amount of concealer with a clean fingertip or brush and blend it out to restore the area.
2. **Dry Brush for Minor Smudges:**
    - For very minor smudges, especially powder fallout, use a clean, dry brush to gently sweep away the residue.

Correcting Over-Applied Blush or Bronzer:

1. **Blend It Out:**
    - If you've applied too much blush or bronzer, use a clean, fluffy brush to blend the product out. You can also use a bit of translucent powder on the brush to help diffuse the color.
2. **Foundation Sponge:**
    - Press a damp makeup sponge that still has a bit of foundation on it over the overdone area. This can help lift some of the pigment and soften the appearance.

Fixing Cakey Foundation:

1. **Mist and Blend:**
    - Spritz your face lightly with a hydrating mist or setting spray, then gently pat the area with a beauty sponge. This can help redistribute the product and eliminate cakey patches.
2. **Add Moisturizer:**
    - Mix a tiny amount of moisturizer with your foundation on the back of your hand and apply it to areas where the makeup has settled or looks heavy. This reintroduces moisture and helps smooth out the texture.

Lipstick Bleeding:

1. **Clean Up with Concealer:**
    - Use a small brush dipped in concealer to outline your lips after applying lipstick. This creates a barrier that prevents color from bleeding and also sharpens your lip line.
    - Set the concealer with a little powder for extra security.

2. **Lip Liner Barrier:**
    - Before applying lipstick, line your lips with a clear or matching lip liner. This not only defines the shape but also helps to keep the lipstick within bounds.

Touching Up Faded Makeup:

1. **Portable Essentials:**
    - Keep essential items like a mini mascara, lip color, and a compact powder in your bag for quick touch-ups. This is especially useful for long days or when transitioning from day to night events.
    - Blotting papers are also handy to remove excess oil without layering more powder.

By mastering these quick fixes, you can ensure that your makeup stays looking fresh and beautiful throughout the day, no matter what minor mishaps might occur. These simple solutions can help you maintain a polished look with minimal effort and disruption to your overall makeup.

Adjusting Your Makeup for Different Lighting

Different lighting conditions can dramatically affect how your makeup looks. What appears perfect in your home may look entirely different under the harsh lights of an office or the dim glow of a restaurant. Understanding how to adjust your makeup for various lighting settings is crucial to maintaining a flawless appearance wherever you go.

Natural Daylight:

1. **Subtle and Soft:**
    - Natural daylight is the most revealing lighting for makeup. Use a light hand, especially with foundation and concealer, to avoid a heavy or cakey appearance.
    - Opt for natural, soft colors for eyeshadows, blush, and lipsticks. Overly bright or dark colors can look too intense in daylight.
2. **Blending is Key:**
    - Ensure all your makeup is well blended. Daylight can highlight any harsh lines or blending mistakes, particularly with contour and blush.

Office or Fluorescent Lighting:

1. **Brighten Your Features:**
   - Fluorescent lighting can wash out your complexion, making you look pale or tired. Choose a foundation that matches your skin tone perfectly and consider a slightly brighter blush or bronzer to bring warmth to your face.
   - Use a highlighter on the high points of your face to bring dimension and light to the skin.
2. **Define Your Eyes:**
   - Enhance your eyes with defined eyeliner and mascara. Under fluorescent lights, eyes can lose some of their impact, so a little extra definition can help.

Evening or Low Light:

1. **Enhance with Colors and Shimmer:**
   - You can afford to go bolder with your makeup in dim lighting. Darker eyeshadows, bolder lip colors, and a bit of shimmer on the eyelids or cheekbones can make your features stand out.
   - Consider using a luminous foundation or adding a drop of liquid highlighter to your base for a glowing complexion.
2. **Stronger Contour and Highlight:**
   - Apply a bit more contour and highlight than you would for daytime. Low lighting can obscure facial features, so enhancing them with contouring and strategic highlights can maintain your face's structure.

Bright Artificial Light:

1. **Mattify Your Complexion:**
   - Bright artificial lights, like those in shops or theaters, can create unwanted shine. Use a mattifying primer and setting powder to keep your skin looking smooth and shine-free.
   - Recheck your makeup under these lights if possible, as you might need additional powder in your T-zone.
2. **Vibrant Lip Colors:**
   - Under bright artificial lights, lip colors can appear washed out. Opt for more vibrant shades that will hold up under strong lighting.

General Tips:

- **Always Check Your Makeup:**
   - Whenever possible, check your makeup in the type of lighting you'll be spending most of your time in. Adjustments might be needed if you move from one type of lighting to another.

- **Carry Essentials for Touch-Ups:**
  - Keep a small makeup bag with essentials like blotting papers, powder, and lipstick for quick touch-ups to adapt to changing lighting conditions throughout the day.

By adjusting your makeup for different lighting conditions, you can ensure you always look your best, regardless of the environment. Understanding these nuances allows you to enhance your natural beauty effectively, keeping your makeup impeccable from sunrise to sunset.

Chapter 14: Advanced Techniques and Trends

Embracing advanced makeup techniques and keeping up with the latest trends are crucial for staying relevant and creative in the world of makeup artistry. This chapter explores innovative ways to apply makeup, experiment with bold looks, and incorporate contemporary trends that can transform your makeup style.

Exploring Colorful Makeup Looks

Colorful makeup offers a fantastic avenue for creativity and personal expression. This section focuses on how to effectively incorporate vibrant colors into your makeup routine, whether for everyday wear or special occasions.

Eye Makeup with Color

1. **Choosing Colors:**
   - **Color Wheel Insights:** Use the color wheel as a guide to select shades that complement your eye color or contrast beautifully for a striking effect.
   - **Trendy Shades:** Keep an eye on current trends for inspiration—neon, pastel, and jewel tones are often popular choices that can be adapted for different looks.
2. **Application Techniques:**
   - **Pop of Color:** For a subtle introduction to colorful makeup, add a pop of color along the lower lash line or as an eyeliner.
   - **Colorful Crease:** Blend a bright color into the crease while keeping the rest of the eyelid neutral. This adds an element of surprise to your makeup.
   - **Full Lid:** For a more daring look, apply a vibrant shade across the entire lid. Blend out the edges with a neutral shade to ensure a seamless transition.

Blush and Highlighter

1. **Vibrant Blush:**
   - **Bright Blushes:** Choose blushes in bright pinks, corals, or even reds. Apply lightly and blend thoroughly to ensure the color enhances your cheeks without overpowering your face.
2. **Colored Highlighter:**

o **Beyond the Norm:** Explore highlighters in unusual colors like lavender, icy blue, or even light green. These can add a unique glow to your skin, especially in themed makeup looks or creative projects.

Lip Colors

1. **Bold Lip Choices:**
   - o **Statement Lips:** Don't hesitate to try bold lip colors. Vibrant oranges, hot pinks, or deep purples can transform your look dramatically.
   - o **Ombre Lips:** For a more advanced application, try an ombre lip using two complementing bold colors, blending them together where they meet.

Integration Tips

1. **Balance Your Look:**
   - o When incorporating bold colors, keep the rest of your makeup more subdued to let the colors stand out without clashing.
   - o Decide on one feature to emphasize with color (eyes, lips, or cheeks) and keep the others neutral.
2. **Wearable Art:**
   - o Colorful makeup doesn't just have to be for special occasions. Integrate small elements into your everyday makeup, like switching your regular black eyeliner for a vibrant teal or using a tinted lip balm in a bold color.
3. **Layer and Blend:**
   - o Layering different shades and blending them well is key to achieving a sophisticated colorful look. Use a good set of brushes and blend edges for a smooth gradient of color.

Experimentation and Practice

- **Practice Makes Perfect:**
  - o Experiment with different color combinations and placements. Practice different looks in your free time to see what works best for your face shape, skin tone, and personal style.
- **Stay Inspired:**
  - o Follow makeup artists and trends on social media platforms like Instagram and YouTube for continuous inspiration and new ideas.

Colorful makeup is all about fun and self-expression. Don't be afraid to step out of your comfort zone and try new, vibrant looks that showcase your personality and artistic skills.

Experimenting with Bold Lip Colors

Bold lip colors are a powerful tool in makeup artistry, capable of transforming any look from ordinary to spectacular. Here's how to confidently experiment with daring shades and textures to create standout lip looks.

Choosing Bold Lip Colors

1. **Selecting Shades:**
   - **Rich Reds and Vibrant Pinks:** Classic bold colors like deep reds and bright pinks are always in style and suit a variety of skin tones.
   - **Unconventional Colors:** Don't shy away from unusual colors like blues, greens, or even black for a dramatic, edgy look. These can be particularly striking for special events or creative photoshoots.
2. **Understand Undertones:**
   - Pay attention to the undertones in your skin and the lip colors. Warm undertones pair well with warm colors like orange-reds, while cool undertones look great with blue-based reds or purples.

Application Techniques

1. **Preparation:**
   - **Lip Exfoliation:** Start by exfoliating your lips to ensure a smooth surface. Use a sugar scrub or a soft toothbrush to gently rub away any flaky skin.
   - **Moisturization:** Apply a nourishing lip balm and let it absorb for a few minutes before blotting away the excess. This helps the lipstick apply evenly and stay comfortable.
2. **Lip Liner:**
   - **Defining the Lips:** Outline your lips with a lip liner that matches or complements your lipstick. This not only defines the shape but also creates a barrier to prevent the color from bleeding.
   - **Filling In:** Fill in the entire lip with the liner to create a base that will help the lipstick last longer and enhance the color intensity.
3. **Lipstick Application:**
   - **Precision with a Brush:** For bold colors, precision is key. Use a lip brush to apply the lipstick, starting at the center of the lips and working outwards. The brush allows for more controlled application than applying directly from the tube.

- **Building Layers:** Apply one layer, blot with a tissue, and then apply a second layer. This technique builds color intensity and longevity.

Finishing Touches

1. **Check Edges:**
   - Clean up any smudges or uneven edges with a small brush dipped in concealer. This sharpens the edges and makes the lip color pop.
   - Set the concealer with a tiny bit of powder to ensure it stays in place.
2. **Highlight:**
   - Add a dab of highlighter to the cupid's bow and the center of the lower lip. This not only accentuates the lip shape but also gives the illusion of fuller lips.

Longevity and Maintenance

1. **Touch-Up Kit:**
   - Carry your lipstick and a mini mirror for quick touch-ups throughout the day or night, especially after eating or drinking.
   - Include a few cotton swabs and a small amount of concealer for any necessary corrections.
2. **Hydration:**
   - Keep your lips hydrated with lip balm as needed, especially if using matte lipsticks, which can be drying over time.

Experimenting with bold lip colors can be an exciting way to express your personality and enhance your makeup look. With the right preparation, application techniques, and confidence, you can pull off any bold lip with style.

Incorporating Current Makeup Trends

Staying up-to-date with the latest makeup trends allows you to refresh your look and explore new styles. This section covers how to incorporate contemporary makeup trends into your routine, ensuring you remain fashionable and innovative in your makeup application.

Staying Informed

1. **Follow Industry Leaders:**

- Keep an eye on famous makeup artists, influencers, and beauty brands on social media platforms like Instagram, TikTok, and YouTube. These channels are often the first to showcase emerging trends and tutorials.
- Attend beauty expos, subscribe to fashion and beauty magazines, and follow beauty blogs to get insights into upcoming trends and how to execute them.

Trend Examples and How to Adapt Them

1. **Dewy, Glass-like Skin:**
   - Achieve a radiant, hydrated complexion by focusing on skincare. Use products like hyaluronic acid serums, and moisturizers to enhance skin moisture.
   - Apply a luminous foundation and use highlighters strategically on the high points of your face to emulate a dewy glow.
2. **Bold Eyeliner Styles:**
   - Experiment with graphic eyeliner looks, such as floating crease liners or winged eyeliner in non-traditional colors. Practice using a steady hand and consider using stencils or tape to achieve precise lines.
   - Use gel liners or vibrant liquid eyeliners to add a pop of color or create dramatic shapes that draw attention to the eyes.
3. **Vivid and Pastel Eyeshadows:**
   - Embrace color by incorporating vivid or pastel eyeshadows into your look. Start with a neutral base and blend in brighter colors for a gradient effect.
   - For a more subtle approach, apply a wash of pastel eyeshadow on the lids paired with minimalistic face makeup.
4. **Statement Lips:**
   - Bold lip colors can transform your makeup look. Try out different finishes such as matte, satin, or gloss in trending colors like deep plum, bright orange, or classic red.
   - Prep your lips to ensure smooth application and long wear, especially when using matte formulas.

Technique Adaptation for Personal Style

1. **Blend Trends with Personal Aesthetics:**
   - Not every trend needs to be adopted as is. Adapt trends to suit your personal style and comfort level. For instance, if bold lips are in but you prefer subtler makeup, opt for a sheer tint or a lip stain instead of a full-coverage lipstick.

2. **Trial and Error:**
    o Practice at home before debuting a new trend in public. This allows you to adjust the intensity, colors, and techniques to better suit your features and preferences.
3. **Professional Development:**
    o Continuously improve your skills through online tutorials, workshops, and courses. The more adept you become at various techniques, the easier it will be to adapt trends into wearable looks.

Reflecting Current Trends in Everyday Makeup

- **Mix and Match:**
    o Combine elements from multiple trends to create a unique look that remains on-trend but also personal and unique to you.
- **Subtle Integrations:**
    o If you're hesitant about embracing full trend looks, incorporate small elements, such as using just a touch of glitter along the lash line or a subtle hint of neon in your eyeliner.

Incorporating current makeup trends into your routine doesn't mean a complete overhaul of your style. Instead, it's about choosing elements that resonate with you and adapting them in ways that enhance your natural beauty and express your individuality.

Chapter 15: Taking Care of Your Makeup and Tools

Proper maintenance of your makeup and tools is essential not only for hygiene but also to ensure the best application and longevity of your products. This chapter provides detailed guidance on cleaning and organizing your makeup, sanitizing your tools, and knowing when it's time to replace your makeup products.

Cleaning and Organizing Your Makeup

Maintaining a clean and organized makeup collection is essential not only for hygiene but also for efficiency and longevity of your products. Here's how to effectively clean and organize your makeup, ensuring everything is in prime condition and ready to use.

Organizing Your Makeup

1. **Sort by Category:**
   - Divide your makeup into categories such as face, eyes, lips, and tools. This makes it easier to find what you need and streamlines your makeup application process.
2. **Use Appropriate Storage:**
   - Invest in storage solutions like drawers, makeup organizers, or cosmetic bags. These help protect your products from dust and direct sunlight which can degrade the quality of the makeup.
   - Consider the environment: Keep makeup in a cool, dry place away from humidity which can cause products to deteriorate faster.
3. **Frequent Reviews:**
   - Periodically go through your makeup collection to remove expired products or items you no longer use. This helps keep your collection fresh and relevant to your needs.

Cleaning Your Makeup

1. **Exterior Cleaning:**
   - Regularly wipe down the exteriors of makeup products with a damp cloth to remove dust and spills. Keeping the exterior clean helps prevent dirt from transferring to your face or hands during use.
2. **Product Specific Cleaning:**

- o **Lipsticks:** Wipe off the top layer of the lipstick with a tissue soaked in alcohol every few weeks to remove bacteria and keep the product fresh.
- o **Powdered Products:** For compacts and eyeshadows, scrape off the top layer if it develops a hard film or appears shiny, which can be a sign of oil buildup from your brushes.

3. **Sharpenable Items:**
- o Regularly sharpen items like eyeliner and lip pencils. This not only keeps the product fresh but also ensures hygiene as it removes the outer layer that might have been exposed to bacteria.

Hygiene Best Practices

1. **Avoid Double Dipping:**
- o Especially for products used wet, such as mascaras and liquid eyeliners, avoid putting the applicator back into the product after it has touched your skin. This practice can introduce bacteria into the product.

2. **Use Disposable Applicators:**
- o When possible, especially during makeup trials or when someone else uses your makeup, use disposable applicators to maintain hygiene.

3. **Regular Check-ups:**
- o Every few months, do a thorough check of your makeup. Smell products, check textures, and look for any signs of mold or separation, particularly in liquid products.

By keeping your makeup collection clean and organized, you not only ensure better application but also significantly extend the life of your products. This routine also helps prevent skin irritations and infections that can occur from using old or contaminated cosmetics.

Sanitizing Your Tools

Keeping your makeup tools clean is crucial for maintaining skin health and ensuring the best performance of your makeup application. Regular sanitization helps prevent the buildup of bacteria, oils, and product residue that can lead to skin irritations or acne. Here's a comprehensive guide to effectively cleaning and sanitizing your makeup tools.

Daily Cleaning

1. **Brushes and Sponges:**
   - After each use, wipe off excess product on a clean paper towel or a microfiber cloth. This simple step helps prevent color mixing the next day and removes some surface bacteria.
2. **Quick Sanitizing Spray:**
   - Use a quick-drying brush cleaner spray for daily sanitation. Spray directly onto the brush or sponge and gently wipe clean. This will not substitute for deep cleaning but helps keep tools usable between washes.

Deep Cleaning

1. **Weekly Brush Cleaning:**
   - Soak brushes in warm water, then gently massage a brush cleanser or mild soap (baby shampoo works well) into the bristles. Rinse thoroughly until the water runs clear. Avoid getting water into the brush ferrule as this can loosen the glue over time.
2. **Cleaning Sponges:**
   - Soak sponges in warm soapy water, then squeeze and massage them to work out makeup and dirt. Rinse thoroughly until all soap is removed. For stubborn stains, using a sponge-cleaning solution or micellar water can be more effective.

Drying Techniques

1. **Brushes:**
   - After washing, reshape the bristles and lay brushes flat on a towel with the bristles hanging off the edge of a counter. This allows them to dry in their natural shape and prevents water from seeping into the handle.
2. **Sponges:**
   - Squeeze out excess water with a clean towel and leave them to air dry in an open, ventilated space. Ensure sponges are completely dry before storing them to prevent mold and bacteria growth.

Sanitizing Metal Tools

1. **Tweezers, Eyelash Curlers, and Scissors:**
   - Wipe down with rubbing alcohol before and after each use. This is especially important for tools that come into contact with your eyes or any broken skin.
2. **Monthly Deep Clean:**

- For metal tools, consider a deeper clean by soaking them in a disinfectant solution for tools or boiling them for a few minutes to ensure all bacteria are killed.

Maintaining Tool Quality

1. **Storage:**
   - Store tools in a clean, dry place. Consider using protective covers for brushes or keeping them in a separate compartment away from makeup products to avoid cross-contamination.
2. **Replacement:**
   - Regularly inspect tools for wear and tear. Replace sponges every three months, or sooner if they start to crumble or retain odors. Brushes generally last several years but should be replaced if bristles begin to fall out or if they remain stiff after cleaning.

Properly sanitizing and maintaining your makeup tools not only extends their lifespan but also protects your skin from potential irritants and infections. This routine is an essential part of any makeup practice, ensuring that your application is always clean, safe, and beautiful.

When to Replace Makeup Products

Using fresh makeup is crucial for effective application and skin health. Over time, makeup can harbor bacteria, lose effectiveness, or change in texture and smell, which can lead to skin irritation or infections. Here's a guide to knowing when it's time to replace your key makeup products.

Product Lifespan Guidelines

1. **Mascara:**
   - Replace every 3-6 months. Mascara is prone to bacterial growth because the tube provides a moist environment that facilitates bacteria proliferation, and the close contact with the eyes increases infection risks.
2. **Liquid Eyeliner:**
   - Replace every 3-6 months for similar reasons as mascara, especially if it's a formula you dip into a tube.

3. **Foundation and Concealer:**
   - Liquid foundations and concealers should be replaced every 6-12 months. If the product starts to separate, change color, or develop an off smell, it's time to toss it earlier.
4. **Lipsticks and Lip Glosses:**
   - Replace lip products every 12-18 months. If you notice any changes in texture, smell, or if it becomes dry and difficult to apply, replace it sooner.
5. **Powders (Eyeshadow, Blush, Bronzer, Setting Powder):**
   - These can last up to 2 years since powders are less likely to harbor bacteria. However, if you notice any hard film forming on the surface, a change in smell or color, or if they become chalky and less pigmented, it's time to replace them.
6. **Cream Products (Blush, Eyeshadow, Contour Kits):**
   - Cream products should generally be replaced every 12-18 months. They can go bad quicker than powders because they contain more water and oils, which can encourage bacterial growth.

Signs It's Time to Replace

1. **Change in Texture or Consistency:**
   - If a product thickens, dries out, or becomes lumpy, these are clear signs it's past its prime.
2. **Off Smell:**
   - Any change in the way a product smells is a strong indicator of spoilage or bacterial growth.
3. **Irritation:**
   - If using a product suddenly causes your skin to break out, become itchy, or turn red, discontinue use immediately and replace it.
4. **Application Issues:**
   - If the product no longer applies smoothly or the color payoff has diminished, it's likely time to get a new one.

Best Practices for Makeup Longevity

1. **Storage:**
   - Store makeup in a cool, dry place away from direct sunlight to extend its shelf life.
2. **Hygiene:**
   - Wash hands before using products, especially those in pots or pans. Consider using a spatula or a clean brush instead of fingers to avoid introducing bacteria.

3. **Avoid Sharing:**
    o Never share makeup, especially products used around the eyes and lips, to prevent the spread of bacteria and potential infections.

Knowing when to replace makeup products not only ensures better application but also protects your skin from potential harm. Regularly checking and maintaining your makeup collection will keep your makeup routine safe and effective.

Conclusion

As we conclude "Makeup Tutorial for Black Women: Makeup Mastery for Beginners," it's my hope that you have found this guide not only informative but also empowering. We've journeyed together through the essentials of skin care, the art of makeup application, and the nuances of maintaining and elevating your beauty regimen. Each chapter was carefully crafted to help you unleash your true glow, tailored specifically to the unique beauty needs of black women.

From understanding your skin type to mastering advanced makeup techniques, this book aims to equip you with the knowledge and skills to feel confident and beautiful in your skin. We explored everything from the basics of hydrating and priming your skin, to selecting the right shades for foundation, eyes, and lips that complement deep skin tones beautifully. Moreover, we delved into specialized techniques for eye makeup, contouring, and even tips for special occasions, ensuring you're prepared for both daily life and extraordinary events.

Remember, makeup is not just about enhancement but expression. It's a form of self-love and an art that allows you to portray your inner strength and grace on your own terms. I encourage you to keep practicing the techniques discussed, experimenting with new trends, and most importantly, to continue celebrating your individuality through every brush stroke.

Thank you for allowing this book to be a part of your makeup journey. May you continue to shine brightly, showcasing your true glow wherever you go. Whether you're stepping out for a regular day, a special event, or simply enjoying the process of beautification, remember that each moment you spend on yourself is a testament to your worth and beauty.